Twelve Essential Oils of the Bible

Ancient Healing Oils and Their Contemporary Uses

Karin Opitz-Kreher and Johannes Huber

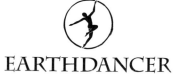

EARTHDANCER

AN INNER TRADITIONS IMPRINT

First edition 2023
Twelve Essential Oils of the Bible:
Ancient Healing Oils and Their Contemporary Uses
Karin Opitz-Kreher and Johannes Huber

This English edition © 2023 Earthdancer GmbH
English translation © 2023 JMS books LLP
Editing by JMS books LLP (www.jmseditorial.com)

Originally published in German as: *Bibelöle, Die Kraftvollen Öle aus der heiligen Schrift*
World © 2015 Schirner Verlag, Darmstadt, Germany

Cover design: DesignIsIdentity.com
Cover illustration: koosen (bowl), Pinci, both shutterstock.com

Typesetting: Chris Bell, cbdesign
Typeset in ITC Garamond
Printed and bound in China by Reliance Printing Co., Ltd.

Cataloging-in-Publication Data for this title is available from the Library of Congress.

ISBN 978-1-64411-765-1 (print)
ISBN 978-1-64411-766-8 (ebook)

Published by Earthdancer, an imprint of Inner Traditions
www.earthdancerbooks.com, www.innertraditions.com

Contents

Introduction

Working with essential oils, with all their active ingredients, is like entering a different universe and discovering a whole new world. How do they work? Which oil is best to use when? Which oils work most effectively on a physical level and which have emotional or mental health benefits? What uses does a particular oil have? What distinguishes one essential oil and its active ingredients from another? What is the chemistry of each oil? Which oils feature in the Bible? The more you explore and engage with such questions, the more you learn and the more you become immersed in ancient wisdom. New horizons await discovery and your own experiences are key, as one by one you explore the oils and discover their particular qualities.

In order to grasp the full potential of biblical or anointing oils, we must go back to ancient scriptures and study the plants themselves. These oils offer us so much more than just the pleasant fragrances such as cedarwood or sandalwood that are used in the perfume industry.

Knowing how the oils were used centuries ago will reveal their power and allow us to make the fullest use of their properties in the present.

Imagine traveling back to a long-forgotten age. Cave paintings discovered in the Dordogne in Southwest France dated to around 15000 BCE reveal how our ancestors used plants as medicine. Aromatic oils manufactured in Egypt as long ago as 4500 BCE were used for ritual purposes or as perfumes, cosmetics, and medicine.

Knowledge of these precious essences is a millennia-old tradition, and skill at working with them is highly prized once more today. A paper by Dr. Manfred Doepp suggests that oils such as frankincense or myrrh provide protection against electromagnetic pollution and can reharmonize the pituitary gland and the hypothalamus. Both are of great relevance in today's world in which cell phones, wifi, and games consoles, and the radiation that they emit, surround us and "switch" our brains. This can lead to addictive behaviors, when after exposure to electromagnetic pollution, for example, the brain can no longer distinguish between what is beneficial or harmful to it. We see how dependent our children and young people are on their various devices and how important it can be to take protective measures (such as applying oils), particularly with young bodies that are still developing.

We wanted to see for ourselves the effects that electromagnetic pollution has on our energy field. Using chakra and aura visualizations, we were able to see how a stable energy field collapsed when a phone number was dialled on a cell phone; the greatest transmission energy, and therefore the highest radiation exposure for the user, is emitted during dialling. When essential oils were used at the moment of exposure to the radiation, we could see how the energy field stabilized once more.

Medicinal Plants and Essential Oils

in Evolutionary and Biblical History

We shall attempt to do justice to all the many scientists, historians, and biblical Christians in the world as we examine the oils from a range of different perspectives.

THE EVOLUTION OF PLANTS AND ESSENTIAL OILS

Join us on a journey through the history of planet Earth that will bring us up to the present day. This excursion into evolution is key to our understanding of how, over time, essential oils have developed into such powerful allies.

We embarked upon this very same journey through time in a lecture given by Dr. Kurt Schnaubelt in Vienna in September 2013, and we hope to share our insights with you. Try to imagine the planet forming billions of years ago, when all that existed were molecules interacting with one another. The first structures began to form, after which the first chromosomes began to evolve. The basic building blocks of life are approximately 3.5 billion years old, while the first living creatures appeared in water some 2 billion years ago.

Several million years ago, the first more complex organisms appeared on land, in coastal regions and on shorelines. These were the "pioneer plants," exceptionally hardy species that were particularly adept at adapting to their circumstances. The plantlife of the time included ginkgo and horsetail which became established on land, but since these primordial plants were preceded by the development of viruses, bacteria, and fungi, they developed essential oils (also known as secondary plant compounds) as a means of protection. If the oils proved effective, then the plants survived.

Insects arrived several hundred million years later and plants continued to develop. The essential oils were now produced not only to protect the plant but also to attract insect life. Angiosperms evolved, plants with a perianth, a structure enclosing the calyx and the corolla (the sexual organs). Over many years, plants developed a highly complex intelligence system for their own protection, and those that are still around today have evolved potent and effective essential oils that have helped them to survive.

We now seek to use reason and science to strip essential oils down to their constituent parts, and the more powerful the measuring instruments we use to explore and assess their properties, the better we succeed. This provides answers to questions about how and why the oils work. We now know a great deal about them and yet they still retain an air of mystery. Each essential oil comprises a whole host of organic molecules, but it is the harmony in the nature of the composition of each particular oil that makes the subtle distinction between whether it is greatly effective or not. To use the metaphor of music, it is the combination of the various instruments in an orchestra that produces a superb symphonic sound, not just a single violin.

A BIBLICAL PERSPECTIVE

At the beginning of St. John's Gospel we read: "In the beginning was the Word, and the Word was with God, and the Word was God. The same was in the beginning with God. All things were made by him; and without him was not any thing made that was made."

That is why plants, as forms of life, can serve us so well, whereas manmade substances, whether synthetic oils or other materials, do not have the same effect. We should return to Nature once more and harness its power, as we too are part of Nature. The environmental physician Klaus-Dietrich Runow explains that our contemporary lifestyle brings us into contact with many of the 80,000 registered artificial chemicals that exist in our modern world, including softening agents in plastics, parabens in cosmetics, pesticides, solvents, and heavy metals.

The human body can absorb a great deal, but like a barrel brimming with liquid, at some point it may overflow, revealing its burden in the symptoms of disease or neurological illness. We tend to associate Parkinson's, Alzheimer's, or MS (multiple sclerosis) with older people, but, shockingly, increasing numbers of young people are also being affected by these conditions. The time has come to rethink our behavior and to make a conscious decision about what we allow to be near us and to enter our bodies.

Consider this. Later in the book we identify how precious anointing oils were used to prepare a body for mummification. Why, today, do we continue to attack our living bodies with poisonous substances?

**Extract from the Creation story in the
Book of Genesis in the Old Testament**

"In the beginning God created the heaven and the earth.
And the earth was without form, and void; and darkness
was upon the face of the deep. And the Spirit of God moved
upon the face of the waters (…). And God said, Let the earth
bring forth grass, the herb yielding seed, and the fruit tree
yielding fruit after his kind, whose seed is in itself, upon the
earth: and it was so. And the earth brought forth grass, and
herb yielding seed, and the tree yielding fruit, whose seed
was in itself after his kind:

and God saw that it was good."

A JOURNEY ACROSS TIME AND THE GLOBE: HOW WE BEGAN USING ESSENTIAL OILS

Plants have been used since time immemorial as a means of nutrition,
for building materials or as medicine. If we take a long leap back
into our history, we see how humans developed from being hunter-
gatherers to farmers and keepers of livestock, and with this change in
way of life came new challenges.

Agriculture and animal husbandry were common practice, and
proximity to animals meant that people were also at risk of illness
and contracting diseases such as plague. Unclean water caused cholera and typhus, while insects attracted to human settlements also
transmitted a range of diseases. We see parallels in the Bible in the
accounts of plagues of insects and diseased livestock.

It was during this period that many animals were also sacrificed
in the temples. This slaughter of beasts in the heat, combined with

the smell of burning flesh and feathers, created an unpleasant stench. To sweeten the atmosphere in the temples therefore, and to protect from disease, herbs and resins were burned as incense and fresh herbs would be scattered across the floor, releasing their scent when trodden underfoot.

Thanks to the way plants evolved to respond to the demands and challenges of their environment by producing essential oils as a protective mechanism, plants came to our aid. People began to exploit their particular qualities, making use of the essential oils' nutritious, protective, cleansing, oxygenating, and regenerative properties. Their inherent power was recognized and used in a host of different ways. The elite—the rulers and priests—used the essential oils in the form of precious distillates, which had a much more powerful effect than the fresh or dried herbs used by the general public.

Evidence for the use of plants for medicinal purposes and their systematic cultivation has been found in the cuneiform writings of the advanced civilizations that flourished around the Euphrates and Tigris rivers, in Western Asia. King Marduk-apla-iddina (772–710 BCE) grew herbs for medicinal purposes in his gardens in Babylon, including plants such as fennel, myrrh, garlic, caraway, and poppy.

Trade routes for spice merchants were established between the Mediterranean region and Jordan, and the Bible's Promised Land saw the use of medicinal herbs and essential oils from Arabia, Lebanon, Persia, Southeast Europe, Egypt, Libya, India, Indonesia, and the Himalayas. This exchange of precious commodities and goods was accompanied by the dissemination of medical knowledge and healing methods.

Essential oils and plants that produce aromatic oils are mentioned as many as 1,035 times in the Bible, and at least 33 plant species are recorded, including frankincense, myrrh, sandalwood, juniper, caraway, galbanum, calamus, mustard, rose, pine, cedar, cypress, laurel, onycha, wormwood, coriander, aniseed, and myrtle.

Virgin olive oil is frequently mentioned in the Bible, a fatty carrier oil that also contains an aromatic and essential component. It provided a source of nutrition, was used as fuel to light fires, and also served as a base for salves and healing oils. Olive oil of the highest quality from a farmer's own harvest was also given as a tithe (a tax, usually a tenth of a farmer's produce) to the priests.

Ancient Egypt was a key producer and user of essential oils. The *Ebers papyrus*, a well-preserved document containing a compilation of medical texts from the era, dating back to around 1550 BCE, was discovered by Egyptologist and writer Georg Ebers (1837–1898). The scroll, a total of 65ft (20m) in length, features precise observations about symptoms and diagnosis, and lists 877 treatment recipes and their applications. Essential oils were made from the wood, resin, flowers, leaves, roots, and fruits of various plants in Egypt, and in some cases also from oils themselves. The distillation method used was slow and was carried out at low temperatures; it was so gentle that the molecular chains were preserved in their entirety.

This process creates an oil formed of very small oil molecules, free of fat molecules yet with great penetrative ability. It is fascinating to see how some contemporary companies are reviving this ancient knowledge once again today. In ancient Egyptian times these oils formed part of the so-called "medicine of the pharaohs" that was used in the process of mummification.

Mummification

In ancient Egypt, pharaohs and high-status individuals were mummified after death. The body was carefully washed and the brain removed through the nostrils, after which an anointing oil made of resins, beeswax, and aromatic oils was poured into the skull. The left side of the body was then cut open and the embalmer removed some internal organs, usually the liver, lungs, stomach, and intestines. After a special cleansing procedure, these were stored in containers known as canopic jars dedicated to the four Sons of Horus.

The abdominal cavity was cleansed with aromatic oils and palm wine and filled with powdered myrrh. A drying phase followed, using sodium bicarbonate to draw moisture from the body to prevent decay. Only then could the actual embalming begin.

After further washing, heated anointing oil was poured into the body and rubbed into the skin, making it supple. The abdominal cavity was filled with preservative resins, oils (including frankincense, cedar, and myrrh), and spices, which were mixed with beeswax (and sometimes with sawdust) to prevent the abdomen from collapsing. Cloth soaked in anointing oils was sometimes inserted into the nostrils. Once the fingers had been wrapped in thin bands of cloth and the abdomen sealed, for example with wax, or in the case of prominent individuals, a thin sheet of gold, the embalmed corpse was wrapped in linen bandages "glued" in place with resins. Depending on the deceased's status and the substances used, the price for this procedure varied. As well as the Egyptian rulers and their spouses, animals were also mummified, including cats as an act of devotion to the cat goddess Bastet.

The power of plants and oils for physical, mental, and emotional cleansing was known in ancient times, when essential oils were also used to lift the spirits or to protect against disease. Images found in ancient temples depict some of the rituals involving oils, accompanied by chanting and cleansing. The classic anointing oil of the Bible is a mixture of myrrh, cinnamon, calamus, cassia, and olive oil (Exodus 30:23–25). It was used by priests for ritual purposes but not by members of the general public, which would have been considered blasphemous.

In Europe, Greek physician Pedanius Dioscorides (circa 40–90 CE) wrote *De materia medica*, a work describing around one thousand medicinal substances (including 813 of herbal origin, 101 animal-based, and 102 mineral-based), along with 4,740 possible applications. It was seen as the foundation of Western medicine until the 17th century, making him the author of the first serious volume of its kind in Europe. Dioscorides served as a military doctor under the Roman emperors Nero and Claudius and was the greatest pharmacologist of his time.

In ancient Rome, oils were used to cleanse political buildings and temples and were also applied in steam baths to reinforce the immune systems of the bathers.

A similarly long tradition in the use of essential oils, pastilles made from herbs, salves, and perfumes evolved in France, supported by Mary Magdalene, who was a disciple of Jesus and had witnessed his crucifixion. Mary, who had considerable knowledge of healing herbs and oils, settled in France after Jesus' death. According to the *Legenda aurea* (Golden legend), a popular religious text that was widely read until the late Middle Ages, she is said to have been sent to sea with other Christians in a boat with no sails, finally reaching France, where for the next thirty years she spread the knowledge of plants.

In esoteric circles, it is believed that Mary Magdalene, trained in the use of essential oils, ritually anointed the feet of Jesus with precious spikenard oil before his crucifixion, and then dried them with her hair. However, biblical Christians believe that the anointing with spikenard oil was carried out by another Mary, the sister of Martha (John 12:3), whose brother Lazarus was resurrected by Jesus. Once she had arrived in France, Mary Magdalene, who is often depicted in portraits with a container of oil, settled in Saintes-Maries-de-la-Mer. Relics held at the basilica in St. Maximin-la-Sainte-Baume, farther inland in Provence, are said to belong to Mary.

Knowledge of oils from ancient Egypt reached the Celts in France, who were also well versed in the healing power of plants. The Celts revered trees and considered them to have special powers, particularly the elder, oak, ash, willow, hazel, birch, pine, and cedar. This knowledge of medicinal plants, herbs, and oils was passed on from master to pupil but was available only under particular circumstances to the common people.

Hildegard of Bingen (1098–1179), also known as Saint Hildegard, left behind a vast treasure trove of holistic knowledge in the fields of medicine, music, religion, ethics, and cosmology. She wrote several treatises, including *Causae et Curae* (Causes and Cures), a work on the origins and treatment of various diseases, along with *Liber subtilitatum diversarum naturarum creaturarum* (Book of subtleties of the diverse nature of creatures and plants). She was greatly respected during her lifetime and was consulted by many prominent people.

In Europe, it was generally wise women who passed on their knowledge of herbs and oils from generation to generation, including formulations for boosting fertility or indeed terminating pregnancies. To those who knew nothing of the use of plants and herbs, this must have looked like magic, and herbalist women were soon turned into "witches." The first witch burning probably took place in Toulouse

(France) in 1272, a brutal practice that reached fever pitch in the 17th century, with knowledge of oils and herbs almost dying out as a result.

René-Maurice Gattefossé (1881–1950), a French chemist, is considered the father of aromatherapy as we know it today. One particular experience left its mark on him. After receiving serious burns in an explosion in his laboratory, he tried treating them with pure lavender oil and was able to witness at first hand, on his own body, how quickly his wounds healed. Gattefossé went on to train Marguerite Maury (1895–1968), who wrote books on youth, beauty, and health with essential oils, and Jean Valnet (1920–1995), who achieved extraordinary results as a doctor with his use of essential oils after surgery during the First Indochina War (1950–1952).

Essential oils were also in use in Asian culture. A tract on healing herbs, *Shennong bencao jing* (Herbal classic of the "Divine Farmer" Shennong) was written as early as 2800 BCE and it still forms the basis for books of Traditional Chinese Medicine (TCM) to this day. It was traditionally attributed to the "Divine Farmer" Shennong, a mythical Chinese emperor. This ancient treatise deals with agriculture and the medicinal benefits of many healing herbs. The Ayurveda (Indian traditional medicine system) also records a deep understanding of the effects of plants and oils, and Tibetan medicine similarly features a sophisticated approach to health in which herbs, oils, and minerals are used in treatments.

Nature's powers have been successfully harnessed by many cultures around the globe, and the use of anointing oil and incense during rituals and high church masses has long been part of Western Christian culture.

Due to the links between our own culture and the Bible, this book focuses on how medicinal plants were used and their essential oils were extracted in biblical times. While the extraction methods are not described in the Bible, they can be found in other historical texts.

EXTRACTION METHODS

Fresh plants

Not all plants yield essential oils that can be used as described in this book, but they may still boast healing properties—medicinal mushrooms are a good example. The concentration of essential oils in fresh plants only amounts to around 1–2 percent. Taking fresh plant sap as an example, all the properties are contained in the sap, but the proportion of essential oil is very low.

Freshly cut herbs such as peppermint and marjoram would be brought into temples and laid on stone floors. As people stepped on them, the oil was released, cleansing and refreshing the air.

Dried herbs

Dried herbs contain the high molecular weight components of the plant in concentrated form, although up to 95 percent of the original essential oils evaporates during drying. The advantage of dried herbs lies in their ability to be stored for lengthy periods, during which time they remain in a kind of dormant state. They can be crumbled and stored in an airtight container, and then rehydrated and revived, ready to use in a tea for example.

Steam distillation

The distillation process delivers a concentration of a plant's essential oil by between 50 and 2,000 times. In the case of distillates of rose or Melissa, this can rise up to 5,000 times, making distillates particularly potent. Each drop is precious. Steam distillation was used in Babylon, China, India,

Egypt, and by the Sumerians as long ago as 3500 BCE. One of the oldest oils to be manufactured in this way is cedarwood oil, followed later by distillates of frankincense and myrrh. These pure and concentrated aromatic essences were mixed with a carrier oil before use.

Maceration

During the maceration process, plants are placed in a vessel and a fatty, heavy oil is poured over them to release their fat-soluble components. The Egyptians preferred castor oil for this purpose, although animal fats from geese, cows, hippos, and crocodiles were also used. The Israelites, on the other hand, would use goat fat and olive oil. A popular technique involved warming the oil and then pouring it over the plant matter, which would then be left to macerate for days or weeks before being filtered through sheets of linen. If the oil was still too weak, new plant material could be added, and the process would begin again until the anointing oil reach the desired concentration. Maceration produced an oil mixture that was already diluted and could be used for anointing, massage, or medicinal applications. The essences of very delicate plants such as jasmine were extracted by cold maceration as they cannot tolerate heat and would otherwise be destroyed during the process.

Pressed oils

In biblical times, olive oil was extracted as a pressed oil by applying pressure to the fruit. All citrus essential oils are extracted from the peel of the fruit and are pressed oils. Citrus fruits were not introduced to Europe and the Middle East until around 1000 CE. This explains why lemons are not mentioned in the Bible. Citrus fruits were cultivated in China 4,000 years ago.

Enfleurage

The pressing of oils was not the preferred technique in the biblical era. Instead, a combination of maceration and pressing was used, involving immersing rose petals (for example) in oil and rolling them with a heavy stone. The weight of the stone released the precious aromatic oils from the petals, thereby speeding up the process of oil extraction. This process is known as enfleurage.

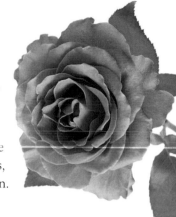

Infusion

The technique of infusion was also based on maceration. Plant material was immersed in oil and then heated, either over a fire or in the sun. This accelerated the release of the fat-soluble essential oils. Fats that had a solid consistency at room temperature were preferred for processing in this manner, which produced a salve once they had cooled.

Rose oil

Time and again throughout history, the knowledge of obtaining oil through steam distillation has been lost. One such period occurred around 500 CE. It was not until centuries later that the Persian physician and scientist Avicenna (980–1037) rediscovered the distillation process and began to specialize in the manufacture of rose oil and rose hydrosol. The distilling equipment of the time was made from clay or stone, materials that are neutral from a chemical perspective and do not react with the oils. Distillation of rose oil is still practiced in the Arabian region.

Incense

Incense such as myrrh, onycha, frankincense, and galbanum was burned in censers (ventilated containers) to disinfect rooms, a common practice in biblical times. It was also burned in temples to create a reverential atmosphere and to ward off disease. We read in Exodus 30:34–36 how Moses was commanded to burn incense to protect the people from plague or pestilence. Essential oils, spices, and resins were either heated directly over glowing charcoal in censers, or by placing the oils, spices, or resins on a small platform over the hot coals. The container could be fastened to a chain and swung, a style of incense burning still in use in Roman Catholic churches today.

Another technique used to burn incense was smudging, which involved blowing smoke from smoldering bundles of incense herbs onto a particular area of the body for therapeutic purposes. Incense was also employed for energetic cleansing along the spine, continuing over the head and down to the feet. This kind of incense burning was particularly popular in India, where it is a practice that continues today. Targeting specific areas of the body by blowing medicinal incense onto them was also practiced by the Egyptians, Greeks, and Romans, and by shamans from South America.

Midwives would place hot coals under the beds or birthing chairs of pregnant women to envelop them in a calming haze of smoke, and supportive myrrh resin was burned to help the mothers-to-be to prepare for delivery and to ease the birthing process.

Moxibustion

During the moxibustion process, mugwort leaves were formed into small cones and burned on or close to the skin at specific acupuncture points as a general restorative treatment. This technique was used as a method of healing in TCM as far back as 140 BCE, and it remains in use today. Knowledge of healing reached Europe via the important trading route of the Silk Road.

We recommend *Healing Oils of the Bible* by Dr. David Stewart and Holger Grimme for more detailed information on extraction methods.

THE QUALITY OF OILS

We take a look in detail at some of the essential oils mentioned in the Bible later in the book, but first a few words to help you make more informed decisions when choosing which essential oils to buy.

Today only a few manufacturers still produce essential oils retaining all their active ingredients. Certain conditions must be met and processes followed, from the sowing, cultivating, and harvesting of the plants, through to distillation, in order to produce an original oil that also preserves the complete chemistry of the plant. Only the highest quality oils will benefit the user, raising the harmonious vibration of their energy field. These complete oils possess a holistic spectrum of effects on all levels—physical, emotional, and spiritual—and are the high-quality oils that we refer to in this book.

A drop of essential oil can contain up to 40 million trillion molecules, a number so vast that it is hard to comprehend. According to Dr. David Stewart and Holger Grimme, just 1 drop of essential oil contains enough molecules to cover every cell in our bodies (around 100 trillion in total) with 40,000 molecules. Once you know that just a single molecule is all that is needed, after it has recognized and bound to its corresponding receptor on a cell, to communicate with the cell's DNA and trigger a change in the cell's function, you will see why even inhaling a small amount of essential oil vapor may have profound effects on the body, brain, and emotions.*

---

* Cf. Stewart, Dr. David; Grimme, Holger: *Healing Oils of the Bible*, Care Publications, 2003, p. 43.

CATEGORIZING OILS

Essential oil is not a protected term and they are not currently certified or approved by any regulatory body in the US. Oils are generally subdivided into the different categories described below.

Pure, natural oils
These are essential oils extracted directly from the plant, resulting in a 100 percent pure essential oil. The label should indicate:

- the plant from which the oil was extracted (plant of origin)
- the relevant part of the plant that is used—root, fruit, peel, petals, leaf
- the chemotype of the plant—the natural composition of the oil (for example, linalool, limes . . .)
- the batch number, which can be used to request a biochemical and physical analysis from the manufacturer

The information given does not include how the steam distillation process, among others, is carried out, which may be rapidly at a high temperature or a more slowly at a low temperature. The oil could well be a 100 percent pure oil of high quality, but this does not necessarily mean it has any therapeutic potency.

Essential oils retaining all their active ingredients
These oils are all natural, 100 percent pure essential oils, extracted directly from the plant and featuring additional indicators of quality.

Cultivation: The plants are grown from seed, which makes them hardier than plants cloned from a mother plant, and in soils that have never been treated with artificial fertilizers. The conditions in which the plants are grown are also important. Plants that are cultivated away from larger cities and industrial areas, therefore minimizing contact with the pollutants of modern-day living, and without the use of pesticides or herbicides, produce better quality oil. I visited the lavender harvest in Provence in southeastern France in 2014 (writes Karin Opitz-Kreher) and saw how they combat pests by spraying the lavender that is attacked by a particular beetle with a liquid mixture containing clay; this deals with the pests without the use of any chemicals.

Harvest: The plants are picked when they reach perfect maturity. This means that they are not necessarily picked at the most economically advantageous time but instead when they are at their peak in terms of quality. The mental attitude of the pickers can also influence the end results. For example, if there are disputes between the workers during the harvest, the result can be measured energetically—the oil harvested under these conditions will not have the same high energetic frequency as oil produced in an atmosphere of harmony. This is supported by observations documented by the Japanese researcher Masaru Emoto (1943–2014) on how words, music, and thoughts can influence water or our blood and form harmonious or disharmonious crystals. Essential oils are like the blood of plants, so it makes sense that these too may react to harmonious or destructive energies. The length of time between the harvesting and the distillation process varies to allow the plant to consolidate its active ingredients. Some plants are left for days before being distilled into the best possible oil, while others are left for years—palo santo, for example.

Distillation: The distillation process plays a key role in facilitating the production of an essential oil that retains all its active ingredients. Distillation is carried out slowly, at low temperatures, and with little pressing. The length of distillation and the temperature at which it is carried out depend upon which plant and which parts (petals, resins, bark, roots) are being processed.

This approach, paying careful attention to the best possible methods to produce the best possible oil, differs from oil produced on a mass commercial scale and is something to take into account if you are offered an allegedly high-value oil at a significant discount. Quality comes at a price.

Natural oils
These oils consist of a range of natural components but are not produced from a single plant. They must not contain synthetic additives.

Natural/nature identical oils
These are a mixture of natural oils and synthetic oils.

Nature-identical oils
These mimic a pure natural oil but have been recreated synthetically and are considerably less complex in their structure. They have a similar scent. A pure, natural rosemary essential oil contians around 150 individual ingredients, but a synthesized, nature identical oil will have only 10–15 components.

Synthetic oils
These do not mimic a natural oil but instead are so-called "designer oils" that have been created to meet specific notions of scent. Very little of their content is natural and they may even be harmful to health.

THE CHEMICAL COMPONENTS OF ESSENTIAL OILS

The bouquet of essential oils consists of many different chemical components, which are composed of carbon, hydrogen, or oxygen. There is a mistaken belief that a plant's individual active ingredients can be isolated in order to achieve optimal results. It is the combination of bitter compounds, enzymes, tannins, mucins, saponins, lecithins, minerals, and the essential oils of a plant that produces its potency, so a full, round, harmonious, and true scent can only be produced when all these components are present.

Carrying out a scent test to compare oils of differing qualities can be very interesting. Once you have experienced the scent of the highest quality oils, others can seem flat, unpleasant, or even pungent.

Now let's take a closer look at the most important chemical bonds in oils for a better understanding of the efficacy of essential oils.

Phenols and phenylpropanoids

Phenols and phenylpropanoids are organic chemical compounds mostly found in cloves, cassia, basil, cinnamon, oregano, aniseed, and peppermint. Some of these are also hot oils, so-called as they can cause the skin to become red, accompanied by a warming sensation, although peppermint is considered hot by some and cooling by others. Phenylpropanoids destroy harmful viruses and bacteria but not beneficial bacteria, which they help to support. Oils rich in phenylpropanoids recognize and open up receptors in our cells and bind to them; communication between the individual cells works better if these are cleansed.

Monoterpenes

Monoterpenes provide protection against free radicals and therefore help to keep us healthy at a cellular level. Plants rich in monoterpenes include galbanum, angelica, hyssop, gum rockrose, peppermint, juniper, frankincense, spruce, pine, cypress, and myrtle.

The chemotypes of essential oils

Oils harvested from the same species of plant may have completely different biochemical compositions depending on the locations and climatic conditions in which they are grown. Variations in the conditions may lead the plants to develop different constituent substances, which can only be identified by gas chromatography. These substances may differ widely from one another and the effects of the respective oils may do the same.

The term "essential oil" bears no indication as to its quality and in fact is rather misleading as it refers to volatile essences that are not at all oily; it is a generic term for a host of organic compounds. The majority of these are organic chemical compounds known as terpenes (monoterpenes and sesquiterpenes). A single oil can contain several hundred individual constituent ingredients, including alkanes, phenols, monoterpenes, sesquiterpenes, diterpenes, alcohols, ether, aldehydes, ketones, esters, lactones, coumarins, and furanoids. We recommend Dr. David Stewart's book *The Chemistry of Essential Oils* for those who wish to explore the composition of essential oils in more detail.

The label on an essential oil bottle should identify the plant and its lead compounds. For example: frankincense, 100 percent pure essential oil; natural ingredients: limes, linalool. The batch number and place of manufacture should also be listed. This will enable you to discover if, for example, thymol is listed on a bottle of oregano essential oil, an ingredient that would otherwise tend to be associated with thyme essential oil. It is the various individual components together that deliver the quality of the oil.

Sesquiterpenes

Sesquiterpenes are a class of terpenes. They enrich the blood and cells with oxygen, and may also help to protect DNA. They improve the blood supply to the pituitary gland and hypothalamus, which has a positive effect on the whole body. Oils with high levels of sesquiterpenes include cedarwood, vetiver, spikenard, sandalwood, ginger, black pepper, patchouli, and myrrh. Sesquiterpenes can also be found in smaller amounts in galbanum, onycha, and frankincense.

To sum up, there is better communication between peptides, hormones, and neurotransmitters when the receptors are cleansed with phenylpropanoids, helping to promote homeostasis (the body's self-regulation of its various systems to maintain a healthy balance between its functions). The effects of the ingredients demonstrate how potent and helpful essential oils can be.

In the past, access to essential oils was confined to certain strata of society, but today they are widely available. Genuine, pure, unadulterated oils remain extremely precious, however, and should be used with care and awareness.

In the following pages, we describe in greater detail the oils of the ancient scriptures. We refer to them as "Bible oils," but these plants and their oils are also mentioned in the ancient writings of other cultures, so we also take a look at the traditions of these countries of origin too as we focus on individual oils.

As already described, our knowledge of essential oils and their application has been in existence for many centuries and handed down through the generations. Some of the applications for the oils have yet to be verified, but many such investigations are now being carried out, and some are available to read online at www.pubmed.gov.

To carry out your own research, simply type in "essential oil" and the name of the particular plant (the Latin or English name). The site is a real treasure trove!

Some of the oils in this book are also of note due to their high antioxidant levels or ORAC (oxygen radical absorption capacity) value. The higher this value, the more effective the essential oil is in dealing with harmful free radicals. ORAC values are listed where available.

Applying oils to the soles of the feet and palms of the hand (see "Practical tip" above) has the following advantages:

- Thanks to the absorbent nature of the skin, the oil soon finds its way to every cell of the body. Since the body's reflex zones are located on the soles of the feet and the palms of the hands, it is possible to reach the entire body through these two areas.

- The skin is less reactive at these points compared to, say, the inner arms, and people who have sensitive skin can dilute the essential oils with a carrier oil before applying them to the feet and hands.

- The skin of these areas is highly absorbent, so only 1–2 drops of essential oil are needed to achieve good results. If the oils were applied to the stomach or upper thigh, for example, much larger amounts of oil would be required to achieve a similar effect.

Once the oil has been applied, rub any remaining traces onto the ears, where more reflex zone points are located. Never introduce essential oils into the ear; oils should only be applied externally and massaged into the skin.

Twelve Essential Oils of the Bible

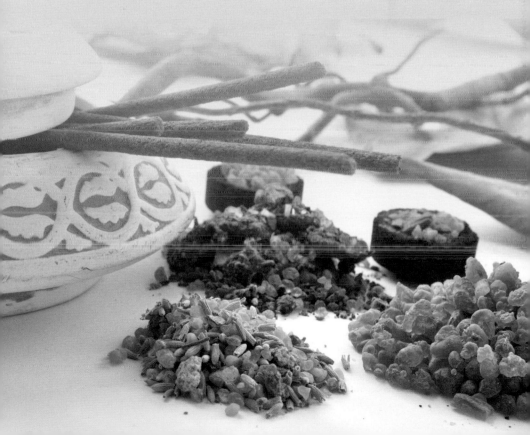

Cassia, Chinese Cassia

(Cinnamomum cassia)

Psalm 45:7-8

"Thou lovest righteousness and hatest wickedness; therefore God, thy God, hath anointed thee with the oil of gladness above thy fellows. All thy garments smell of myrrh, and aloes [sandalwood], and cassia, out of the ivory palaces, whereby they have made thee glad."

CASSIA IN HISTORY

Chinese cassia, also known as Chinese cinnamon, is one of the earliest examples of a spice used for specific treatments and is cited in the *Shennong bencao jing* (see p. 16). It also features in the *Pen Ts'ao*, a comprehensive and classic textbook listing all the plants, animals, minerals, and other substances habitually used in Chinese medicine. This book was written during the Ming Dynasty (1368–1644), although scientific evidence of the effects of the spice had already been established in China as early as the 4th and 3rd centuries BCE. Chinese cinnamon is harvested from the bark of evergreen trees belonging to the laurel family, which can grow to a height of up to 60ft (18m).

Cassia boasts a long biblical tradition. It features as a spice in the Bible under the name *quesiah* and was known in Egypt as a means of containing epidemics of disease, hence the commandment to Moses for the Israelites to take cassia with them, along with myrrh, cinnamon, olive oil, and bulrushes, when they left Egypt. It is also mentioned in one of the oldest medicinal tracts, the *Ebers papyrus* (see p. 12). Cassia was highly prized for its strong antibacterial properties and was also used as incense to purify the air in the temples.

The Greeks and Romans obtained the spice from merchants traveling from Arabia, who refused to give up the secret of its origins. By the 16th century, the search for these origins had reached such a fever pitch that it became one of the principal reasons Portuguese explorers put to sea, leading to their "discovery" of India and Sri Lanka. A century later, the Dutch entered Sri Lanka, then called Ceylon, at the invitation of the Sinhalese, in order to help fight the Portuguese, who by now partly ruled the country. The Dutch secured a monopoly on the cassia trade and remained in Sri Lanka for 150 years. In around 1770, they systematized the cultivation of Chinese cassia, making the spice more accessible and affordable in the West.

Cassia also has aphrodisiac properties, and Roman author and naturalist Pliny the Elder (circa 23–79 CE) lists it in his work *Naturalis historia* (Natural history) as an ingredient in perfume for men. It was also often

Botanical family: Lauraceae (laurel family)

Extraction method: steam distillation of the bark. Cassia has an aroma very similar to that of cinnamon, although they differ greatly in chemical structure.

ORAC: 15.170 µmol TE/100g

Principal components: trans-cinnamaldehyde, trans-0-methoxycinnamaldehyde, coumarin, cinnamyl, acetate used to fragrance bed linen, but the Book of Proverbs contains a warning against women who use it to make their beds enticing! Perhaps this is why cassia essential oil is also one of the "oils of joy."

Today, cassia oil is used to enhance the flavor of candies and drinks and is also popular in oral hygiene products due to its strong antibacterial properties.

Cassia contains approximately 80 percent phenylpropanoids, which is why it is considered a hot oil, defined as having a warming/reddening effect on the skin. It should always be diluted with a neutral oil when applied to the body.

The phenylpropanoids enhance our electromagnetic frequency, which has a positive effect both on a physical and spiritual level.

PROPERTIES

Cassia was valued in popular medicine for the following properties:

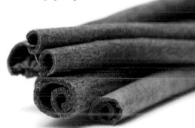

- antibacterial
- antiviral
- antifungal
- anti-inflammatory
- powerfully cleansing

As a hot oil, it provides a pleasantly warming, counteracting effect to the body's reactions to the cold, for example shivering.

Cassia has a strong cleansing effect on an individual's energy field. It is as if the hot fire of cassia can burn away emotional troubles or burdens. Subtle measurements taken of the aura and chakras have revealed how the energy field changes and is cleared once cassia is applied, and how small red flames enter the aura.

POSSIBLE APPLICATIONS

If you have difficulty getting started in the mornings, dilute a neutral oil with a drop of cassia and apply to the soles of the feet, or simply inhale its scent from the oil vial. It is sure to fire up your inner engine!

Daily use

Always dilute 1 part cassia with 4 parts of a neutral carrier oil if it is to come into contact with the skin, and then apply the oil mixture to the chakra points or reflex zone areas.

Use cassia oil undiluted in an ultrasonic diffuser or inhale the scent of the undiluted oil from between the palms of your hands, but be careful as the pure oil can irritate the nasal mucus membrane.

Cassia oil can help you to regain strength if you have pushed yourself beyond your physical limits and are completely exhausted. Apply the diluted oil to the soles of your feet in the morning.

Daily exercise

Do you tend to suffer from cold feet, especially in the chillier months? Take 1 drop of cassia essential oil and dilute it with a neutral carrier oil. Energize the mixture in the palm of your hand (see p. 90) and apply it to the soles of your feet. You will soon feel a pleasant warmth rising up through them.

Galbanum

(Ferula galbaniflua)

Exodus 30:34–35

"And the Lord said unto Moses: Take unto thee sweet spices, stacte [myrrh], and onycha, and galbanum; these sweet spices with pure frankincense: of each shall there be a like weight. And thou shalt make it a perfume, a confection after the art of the apothecary, tempered together, pure and holy."

GALBANUM IN HISTORY

Galbanum is an umbelliferous species of giant fennel. A cut made near the root area produces a rubbery resin. It closely resembles *Ferula foetida*, a plant whose resin is known in Ayurvedic medicine as asafetida and which balances the three *doshas* or humors: *kapha*, *pitta*, and *vata*.

In ancient Egypt, galbanum was used in religious ceremonies and for the process of embalming. Traces of

---

Trade in oils made from galbanum is now no longer permitted as the plant is a protected species, making the oil currently unavailable. Instead, see the Alternative Oil of Elemi on page 87.

Botanical family: Apiaceae or *Umbelliferae* (parsley family)

Extraction method: steam distillation from resin

ORAC: 26.200 μmol TE/100g

Principal components: alpha-pinene, beta-pinene, delta-3-carene, myrcene, sabinene

galbanum have been identified in the cloth wrappings of ancient mummies. The Egyptians also liked to use galbanum as a base oil in a range of perfumes, prizing it for its pleasant scent and therapeutic properties. It was used by the Israelites in salves to treat skin conditions and abscesses, and to heal wounds.

Galbanum is mentioned in the Bible in recipes for incense used for sacred purposes and in offerings to God; its use for profane purposes, on the other hand, was strictly forbidden. Galbanum was also said to offer protection against demons. Greek physician and pharmacologist Dioscorides and Roman author Pliny the Elder both praised its antispasmodic, diuretic, and calming properties, as well as its ability to settle the nerves. As the so-called "mother resin," it helps to boost the female abdominal organs.

According to the Old Testament and ancient Egyptian writings, the plant was highly prized for its medicinal and spiritual properties. It grows particularly well in India and Iran, where the resin is now used in the form of a plaster to treat snake and insect bites. Classical homeopathy also recommends it for rheumatic and similar complaints.

Galbanum oil provides mental support by helping to maintain concentration and boost energy. It can also balance extreme emotions. When used in conjunction with frankincense and sandalwood, it propels the user onto higher frequency planes. The oil is rich in monoterpenes, containing levels of approximately 70–80 percent.

PROPERTIES

Galbanum essential oil was valued in popular medicine for the following properties:

- antiseptic
- mildly antispasmodic
- anti-inflammatory
- stimulates the circulation
- balances digestion
- combats nervous tension
- supports the healing of scars
- invigorates the liver and gall bladder
- generally promotes harmony and equilibrium
- treats bacterial skin problems

Galbanum oil encourages feelings of calm and reduces stress during panic attacks. On an emotional and mental level, it promotes intuition and trust in one's own feelings. It enhances both spiritual awareness and the quality of meditation exercises.

POSSIBLE APPLICATIONS

Apply 2–4 drops of undiluted oil to the desired area and/or to the chakra points or foot reflex zones. It can also be inhaled from between the palms of the hands and/or nebulized in an ultrasonic diffusor.

Daily exercise

The liver is like a large factory in which a vast number of metabolic and hormonal processes take place. One of its roles is to help with the excretion of fat-soluble toxins, hence in today's world it faces considerable challenges posed by our choice of diet and lifestyle. The liver can also be affected by the emotions, which is why slightly grumpy people are sometimes said to be "liverish." To support and relieve the liver, try the following:

Apply 1 drop of galbanum oil directly to the skin over the area of the liver (below the ribcage on the right-hand side). How does the area feel after the application? The relaxing effects can be enhanced by lying down and placing a warm compress on the area. Make this by holding a cloth under warm, running water, squeeze out the excess and place a dry cloth on top of the moist one. Inhaling the scent from between the cupped palms of the hands is also helpful—breathe in the scent deeply.

Myrrh

(Commiphora myrrha)

Esther 2:12

"NOW when every maid's turn was come to go in to king Ahasuerus, after that she had been twelve months, according to the manner of the women, (for so were the days of their purifications accomplished, to wit, six months with oil of myrrh, and six months with sweet odors, and with other things for the purifying of the women)."

MYRRH IN HISTORY

Knotty, thorny myrrh bushes are found in Iran and Libya, on the shores of the Red Sea, and on the coast of Somalia. Myrrh is mentioned in many ancient scriptures, with the earliest references appearing in the ancient Egyptian *Ebers papyrus* (see p. 12). Derived from plant resin, myrrh essential oil has been used for millennia, even dating back some 4,000 years. Myrrh is one of the plants mentioned most frequently in the Bible, along with frankincense and cedar.

The story of Joseph is related in the first book in the Bible, in Genesis 37. He is sold as a slave by his envious brothers to a caravan of traders on their way to Egypt with myrrh and balm. Joseph eventually manages to free himself from slavery and gains the favor of the pharaoh, gradually rising to become the Egyptian governor.

Botanical family: Burseraceae
(incense tree family)

Extraction method: steam
distillation from resin

ORAC: 379.800 µmol TE/100g
https://www.biocrick.com/
Furanoeudesma-1-3-diene-
BCN9925.html

Principal components:
lindestrene, curzerene,
furanoeudesma-1, 3-diene,
methoxyfuronogermacrene,
beta- and gamma-elemene

Many years later, when the brothers visit the governor to ask for food, they do not recognize Joseph, and bring balm and myrrh as gifts (Genesis 43:11), the very same oils that had accompanied him into captivity years before.

Myrrh was well known as a medicine in the ancient world and was used in a number of ways. In Egypt, for example, it was burned as incense and used in sacred ceremonies. Burning the resin was an essential feature of the Egyptian sun cult tradition. A perfume oil known as *kyphi* comprised 16 different essences, one of which was myrrh, while the resin of myrrh was an ingredient in medicinal salves.

In addition to frankincense and gold, the three Wise Men from the East brought Jesus myrrh at his birth. Years later, before his crucifixion, Jesus was offered myrrh in wine on Golgotha, which he refused. Mark 15:23 "And they gave him to drink wine mingled with myrrh; but he received it not." The Israelites would consume myrrh macerated in wine before religious services in order to lift them spiritually, a combination that was also said to ease the fear of death among the dying.

Myrrh was one of the oils used in the embalming process. Nicodemus, described in the Bible as a Pharisee and Jewish leader, provided 100lb (33kg) of myrrh and aloes (sandalwood) to embalm the body of Jesus, a practice customary in ancient times for those who had been revered in life. Myrrh therefore accompanied Jesus both at his birth and after his death. In biblical tradition, myrrh is one of the principal ingredients in anointing oils, along with cedar and sandalwood.

In the Book of Esther 2:12, the Bible details how virgins being prepared for King Ahasuerus of Persia were placed under special care for a year. They were treated with oil of myrrh for the first six months and then with sweet scents for the remaining period. Spices such as sandalwood and cassia were used (see the Bible passage on p. 39). Ahasuerus went on to marry Esther, who through this act of marrige to the king saved her people.

Myrrh is also mentioned in Proverbs 7:17 "I have perfumed my bed with myrrh, aloes [sandalwood], and cinnamon."

Hildegard of Bingen (1098–1179), the Benedictine nun and herbalist, also included myrrh in her compendium of medicine. Myrrh is mentioned in the Qur'an, in the Old and New Testaments, and in Greek and Roman sources. Greek historian Herodotus (circa 484–425 BCE), Greek philosopher Theophrastus of Eresos (circa 371–287 BCE), and Roman author and naturalist Pliny the Elder (23/24–79 CE) classified it as a therapeutic product and cited its use in many recipes for salves. Elixirs for topical applications developed in France all contained myrrh; they were used to treat cuts and burns and to promote the formation of phlegm (in order to expel it). Writing in his *Matière Médicale,* published in 1765, German physician and naturalist Johann Friedrich Cartheuser (1704–1777) describes myrrh as a beneficial treatment against ulcers and other conditions of the skin.

Together with sage, among its other uses, myrrh strengthens the gums. It is one of the most important plants in India's Ayurvedic medicine and plays a central role in oral hygiene and dental health.

Myrrh was also used to treat gynecological issues; the essential oil was applied to the perineum of the mother before giving birth to sterilize the area and help the tissue to stretch. Myrrh oil was also applied to the umbilical cords of babies. In biblical times, the cord was left to fall off of its own accord; this would generally occur after around four days if myrrh oil had been applied, without any accompanying infection or discoloration, instead of the week to ten days that was more usual.

When distilling myrrh essential oil, some conventional manufacturers add ammonia to boost the yield, but this cancels out the oil's potential therapeutic benefits.

The oil is also highly suitable for energetic cleansing for people working with the sick and elderly, and for anyone finding themselves drained of energy and weighed down by the suffering of others. In such cases, myrrh oil helps to keep them on an even keel mentally and boosts their energy field.

Warning: Do not use myrrh essential oil during pregnancy, as it stimulates the womb.

PROPERTIES

Myrrh essential oil was valued in popular medicine for the following properties:

* powerful antioxidant
* anti-inflammatory
* antiviral
* antiparasitic
* antifungal
* anesthetic
* treats tooth and gum infections
* soothes cracked and chapped skin
* helps to plump out wrinkles
* helps to treat stretch marks

Myrrh essential oil is rich in sesquiterpenes; its application balances many vital hormones, including the thyroid and growth hormones. It is also used as a base oil in the perfume industry.

The scent of myrrh oil has a strengthening and stabilizing effect, combating feelings of unease and anxiety. It creates an invisible forcefield around us, a protective cocoon that only allows beneficial energies to penetrate and repels negative energies. The oil can be used in a room spray, for example, to create a protective environment and help keep negativity at bay. It is also very pleasant when added to a warm bath, or emulsified in a natural, chemical-free cream for the skin, honey, or alkali salt. Argan oil is also excellent as a base: add a drop of myrrh essential oil to a little argan oil, rub between the palms of the hands and inhale the scent.

Myrrh essential oil brings inner peace and opens the door to the spiritual world. In terms of its mental health benefits, it is uplifting and can make us more attentive and alert. Using myrrh oil helps to free us from the conditioning of mass consciousness (groupthink) and encourages us instead to live our own lives. It can be applied to the root chakra and helps us to refocus when we feel we are treading water on an emotional or spiritual level. Like frankincense, it also helps to offer protection against electromagnetic pollution.

POSSIBLE APPLICATIONS

Apply 1–2 drops directly to the desired area, or to the chakra points or the foot reflex zones. The scent of the oil can also be inhaled from between the palms of the hands or nebulized in an ultrasonic diffusor.

Daily exercise

When you feel the need to get things under control, apply 1 drop of myrrh essential oil to the nape of the neck, or take a moment to inhale the scent from between your cupped hands and feel your confidence being to grow. With your feet planted firmly on the ground, imagine strong roots extending down from the soles of your feet, anchoring you deep inside the Earth while your head is held erect, as if being pulled upward by a silver thread. Standing tall and invigorated, you will feel grounded but also connected to what lies above, and able to make decisions with renewed momentum.

Myrtle

(Myrtus communis)

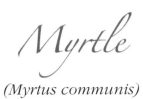

Nehemiah 8:15

"And that they should publish and proclaim in their cities, and in Jerusalem, saying, Go forth unto the mount and fetch olive branches, and pine branches, and myrtle branches, and palm branches, and branches of thick trees, to make booths, as it is written."

Isaiah 55:13

"Instead of the thorn shall come up the fir tree, and instead of the brier shall come up the myrtle tree: and it shall be to the LORD for a name, for an everlasting sign that it shall not be cut off."

MYRTLE IN HISTORY

In ancient Egypt, a concoction of myrtle leaves macerated in wine was used to combat fever and infection. Greek physician Dioscorides (see p. 14) also prescribed it as a fortifying tonic for the stomach for lung and bladder infections. In Greek mythology, myrtle was the favorite plant of the goddess Aphrodite. When she

Botanical family: Myrtaceae (myrtle family)

Extraction method: steam distillation of leaves

ORAC: 25.400 μmol TE/100g

Principal components: alpha-pinene, cineole, limese, linalool

arose, naked, from the waves, she sought shelter behind a myrtle bush on the island of Cythera to shield herself from the lascivious gaze of the satyrs (demons and/or creatures that were half-man, half-beast). In thanks, she granted the myrtle shrub her constant protection.

Myrtle is a symbol of divine, female energy. For the Sumerians (an early civilization that flourished around 3000 BCE in southern Mesopotamia), the myrtle represented the Divine Mother of Heaven.

Myrtle is most frequently characterized as a feminine plant. In the South of France, it was common for women to drink a tisane (infusion) of myrtle leaves to preserve their youthfulness. *Eau d'anges*, a special fragrance containing myrtle leaves manufactured in France in the 16th-century, made use of the plant's toning and astringent (drying excess oils, tightening pores) properties on the skin, while planting a myrtle bush outside the house was said to protect the home from the so-called evil eye.

In biblical times, it was customary for Jewish women to don a wreath of myrtle on their wedding day as a symbol of marital love said to bring good luck. Even today, a combination of myrtle and orange blossom forms part of the wedding finery of a Jewish bride. The French aromatherapy expert Dr. Daniel Penoel has been working in the field of aromatherapy since 1977 and has investigated the effects of myrtle on hormone levels. He has been able to prove that myrtle can rebalance both the thyroid gland and the gonads. Myrtle also has a calming effect on the respiratory system.

PROPERTIES

Myrtle essential oil was valued in popular medicine for the following properties:

- balances the hormonal system (particularly the thyroid gland and ovaries)
- supports the lymph and lung area
- combats sinus infections
- combats throat problems
- treats prostate complaints
- soothes skin conditions (such as acne)
- helps expectoration (coughing up of phlegm)

The liver and hormonal systems are closely connected, allowing the essential oil to support decongestion of the liver while also being supportive on an emotional level in the releasing of feelings of anger and rage. Myrtle essential oil lightens the mood and induces a sense of euphoria. It has a balancing effect on the nervous system and boasts cleansing and invigorating properties. It brings relief from feelings of stress, imbalance, tension, or fear.

On a spiritual level, myrtle oil can underpin our attempts to transcend the ego and instead invest in the belief that we are all one. It balances the masculine and feminine qualities within us, supporting our ability to overcome conflict and regain inner harmony.

POSSIBLE APPLICATIONS

Skin cleansing

Mix 1.5fl oz (50ml) rose water with 5 drops of myrtle oil to cleanse greasy skin. For skin conditions such as severe acne, blend 7 drops of myrtle oil with 2 teaspoons of grape-seed oil, and apply it to the affected areas several times a day.

Mix equal parts of myrtle essential oil with a neutral carrier oil and apply it to the chakra points or foot reflex zones. Inhale it from the palms of your cupped hands or nebulize it in an ultrasonic diffuser.

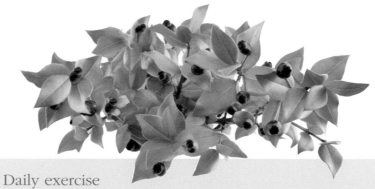

Daily exercise

Try the following exercise when times are challenging or stress-ful and everything feels just too much. Pour a drop of myrtle essential oil into your hand, energize it (see p. 90), and gently massage it into your throat chakra and your back at the sacral chakra. Feel your whole body gradually relax. Applying myrtle oil to the chakras has a powerful effect on the hormonal system. The wheels of energy/chakras of Indian tradition coincide with the location of the body's hormone-secreting glands in Western medical tradition.

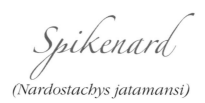

Spikenard

(Nardostachys jatamansi)

Mark 14:3–8

"And being in Bethany in the house of Simon the leper, as he sat at meat, there came a woman having an alabaster box of ointment of spikenard, very precious; and she brake the box, and poured it on his head. And there were some that had indignation within themselves, and said, Why was this waste of the ointment made? For it might have been sold for more than three hundred pence, and have been given to the poor. And they murmured against her. And Jesus said, Let her alone; why trouble ye her? She hath wrought a good work on me. For ye have the poor with you always, and whensoever ye will ye may do them good: but me ye have not always. She hath done what she could: she is come aforehand to anoint my body to the burying."

SPIKENARD IN HISTORY

Spikenard's essential oil produces a calming and relaxing effect. A perennial herb and medicinal plant, in ancient times it was exported to the Mediterranean area from the Himalayas, where it grows at elevations

---

Global trade in oils made from spikenard has now been suspended as the plant is a protected species, making the oil currently unavailable. Instead, see the Alternative Oil of Vetiver on page 85.

of up to 18,000ft (5,500m). Precious salves and oils were made from the rhizome, the rootstock of the plant. Ayurvedic tradition attributes to spikenard consciousness-raising properties and a beneficial effect on the nervous system. It contains high levels (93 percent) of sesquiterpenes. Roman poet Ovid (43 BCE–17 CE) describes how men would anoint their hair with spikenard oil.

Spikenard is also a very precious commodity today, its uncontrolled harvesting in the wild having put it on the list of critically endangered plants. As a result, its export from Nepal is now forbidden. To conserve resources, we recommend very sparing use of spikenard oil and inhalation from the vial by preference.

In the ancient world, where it was reserved for the exclusive use of kings, priests, and initiates, spikenard was one of the most precious of essential oils and was stored in alabaster containers. It was also used by the Israelites and Romans as an oil for anointing the dying.

Various interpretations have been offered of the Bible passage quoted at the beginning of this section, describing how the woman breaks the container to anoint the head of Jesus with the oil, much to the anger of the disciples. They include:

- The woman wished to prepare Jesus for death on the cross.
- She wanted to help Jesus to be better able to forgive the injustice he faced.
- She wished to alleviate his fear of death.

These interpretations of the woman's intentions correspond with spikenard oil's calming qualities and its use in promoting peace and reconciliation. It encourages forgiveness, but the oil can also help to prepare us for when we leave our bodies at the hour of death and return to the higher world. Spikenard encourages us to let go of our fears and master this transition full of trust and with serenity.

Botanical family: Caprifoliaceae
Extraction method: steam distillation of roots
ORAC: 54.800 µmol TE/100g
Principal components: calarene, beta-Ionene, beta-maaliene, aristoladiene

In esoteric circles, it is often said that the anointing of Christ was performed by Mary Magdalene (a supposed sinner), but students of the Bible maintain that it was Mary, sister of Martha and Lazarus. This scene is depicted differently in each of the gospels of Matthew, Mark, Luke, and John: sometimes it is Jesus' feet that are anointed, sometimes his head, and the person applying the oil is not always clearly identifiable. However, no matter who carried out the anointing, it was certainly a gesture of great veneration. The material value of the oil that was used represented about a year's pay for a typical worker of the time.

PROPERTIES

Spikenard oil was valued in popular medicine for the following properties.

- antibacterial
- antifungal
- laxative
- cardiotonic (heart-strengthening)

- antispasmodic
- stomach tonic
- encourages serenity
- releases emotional stress and blockages
- calms the nervous system
- stimulates the secretion of male hormones

The ancient Egyptian priestesses of the goddess Isis worked with spikenard oil as a way of promoting worship of the divine. It is said to have a powerfully calming effect on the dying as they pass to the other side and makes it easier for the soul to leave the body. Spikenard oil is particularly effective when applied to and around the crown chakra.

In order to achieve a cherished goal in this world, we occasionally need a protective shield to fend off negativity and the opinions of others trying to destroy our vision and divert us from our path. Spikenard oil can perform this role, helping to provide protection against negative energies and the taking of criticism too personally. It helps us to work toward our goals with courage and energy.

POSSIBLE APPLICATIONS

Given the endangered nature of plant stocks, we recommend that you inhale the scent of the oil directly from the vial. Spikenard oil can also be diluted with a neutral carrier oil and applied to the chakra points or foot reflex zones, or it can be inhaled from between the cupped palms of the hands.

Applying the oil to a partner can be a relaxing treat for special occasions. Warm a little olive oil and add a couple of drops of spikenard oil. Pour the warmed mixture over your partner's head and they will feel it seeping down through the hair and over the scalp, soaking into the skin. Many people find this a luxurious and emotional experience. The key is to keep the head protected from cold air and drafts after the treatment.

Daily exercise

Is there someone you would like to forgive for the deep hurt they have caused, or has a vexing situation occurred with which you would like to make peace? Take the vial of spikenard oil and inhale its earthy, spicy scent. Picture in your mind's eye the event or person with whom you are not at peace. Put yourself in the other person's shoes and try to see the situation from their perspective. Imagine talking it over with them, or bring the troubling situation to mind and allow feelings of inner peace, understanding, and harmony to flow toward it. Send out love and forgiveness to the person or situation, and to yourself, and feel how a pleasant sense of warmth and peace spreads through your body.

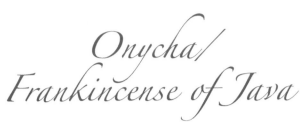

Onycha/ Frankincense of Java

(also known as Styrax benzoin, benzoin, and gum benjamin)

Ecclesiasticus 24:15

"I gave a sweet smell like cinnamon and aspalathus, and I yielded a pleasant odor like the best myrrh, as galbanum, and onyx [onycha], and sweet storax, and as the fume of frankincense in the tabernacle."

ONYCHA IN HISTORY

Onycha, the gum resin of a tree that grows in Java, Sumatra, Malaysia, Laos, and Vietnam, is better known as benzoin but is also sometimes referred to as *Luban Jawi* (frankincense of Java). Onycha arrived in Spain and Italy via Arabia along trade routes, during the course of which its pronunciation changed from *banjawi* to *beijoim* and *belzuri*, and ultimately to *benzoe*, *benzoin* and sometimes *benjamin*. Depending on the preferred Bible translation, the scriptures refer to both onyx or onycha; onyx may also refer to a murex snail living in the Red Sea, but according to the purity laws of the Torah, onycha can only be of vegetable origin since sea creatures without fins and scales were not considered kosher and so could not be used in prestigious rituals.

In 1461, Melech Elmazda, sultan of Egypt, presented the doge of Venice with 30 rotoli of onycha (100 rotoli was the equivalent of 180lb/80kg), along with two valuable Persian carpets. Fifteen years later, he also gave the queen of Cyprus a generous gift of 15 rotoli of onycha.

Botanical family: Styracaceae (silver bells family)

Extraction method: steam distillation from resin

Principal components: cinnamic acid, coniferyl benzoate, benzoic acid, phenylethylene, phenylpropyl alcohols, vanillin

In the ancient world, the oil of onycha was used to treat all kinds of skin conditions and to improve the complexion. It reached Britain in the 16th century and the English became so enamored with its properties that in 1623 they built a factory in Siam (modern-day Thailand) so that they could extract the precious resin themselves.

Nostradamus (1503–1566), the renowned French astrologer, physician, and seer, who published his prophecies in 1555, also listed onycha as an antispasmodic and a skin tonic. It was used in France as a balsam for the lungs, and the resin was burned as incense in the presence of the sick. Small lozenges known as *pastilles du serail* were manufactured as hard candy to counteract colds and influenza.

Onycha essential oil has a balancing effect on the nervous and hormonal systems. Benzoic acid is used as a preservative in the food industry and as an ingredient in the varnish used in making violins. Onycha is also used as a base oil in perfume manufacture. It contains vanillin, which has a delightful scent. No other essential oil (with the exception of vanilla essential oil) contains vanillin, making onycha particularly precious.

It is a good protective oil on a spiritual level, opening up the planes of the heart and crown chakras.

PROPERTIES

Onycha was valued in popular medicine for the following properties:

- antiseptic
- anti-inflammatory
- kind to the skin
- antispasmodic
- helps to heal wounds
- enhances mood
- relaxing
- aphrodisiac
- sensual
- induces feelings of euphoria
- improves the intellect

Warning: Benzoin can produce an allergic reaction.

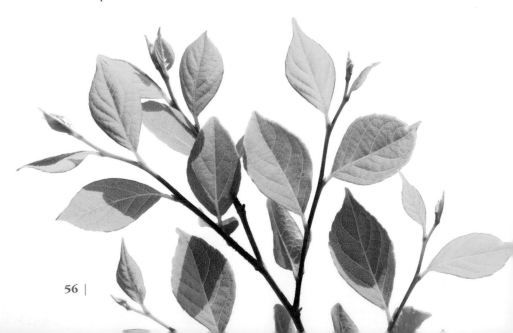

Onycha delivers a sense of safety and protection, and is particularly useful for dealing with feelings of irritability and frustration. It also helps us to cope in times of grief.

POSSIBLE APPLICATIONS

Apply 1–2 drops directly to the chosen area, the chakra points, or reflex zones. Onycha essential oil can also be inhaled from the cupped palms of the hands or nebulized in an ultrasonic diffusor.

Daily exercise

If it feels as though things are getting on top of you and you are being pulled in all directions, try the following: mix 1 drop of onycha oil with a little carrier oil and apply to the ear reflex zones. Rub it in gently (being very careful not to allow any of the oil to enter the ear canal). Inhale the scent from between your cupped hands and take a moment to feel how a sense of warmth, calm, and security spreads through your body.

Sandalwood

(Santalum album)

The Gospel according to John 19:39–40
"And there came also Nicodemus, which at the first came to Jesus by night, and brought a mixture of myrrh and aloes [sandalwood], about an hundred pound weight. Then took they the body of Jesus, and wound it in linen clothes with the spices, as the manner of the Jews is to bury."

SANDALWOOD IN HISTORY

Sandalwood was known as aloes in biblical times (not to be confused with aloe vera). It was an ingredient in anointing oils, along with cedar and myrrh.

There is a long tradition of using sandalwood essential oil in Ayurvedic, Chinese, and Egyptian cultures. The oil was used in religious rituals such as the embalming of the dead, while its wood was carved to create icons representing deities and items for temples. Many different uses are recorded in Indian Ayurvedic tradition, whether for its antipyretic (fever-reducing) qualities, its invigorating properties, or as a remedy for skin rashes, abscesses, and tumors, for which it was worked into a paste. Indian pharmacopoeias also suggest its effectiveness at inducing perspiration (diaphoretic) and as an expectorant.

After the crucifixion of Jesus, the Pharisee Nicodemus and Joseph of Arimathea donated 100lb (45 kg) of sandalwood and myrrh to embalm his body (see the Bible passage at the beginning of this section). The modern equivalent in value would be 110–150,000 US dollars (100–140,000 euros), so it is clear that this was a very extravagant gesture, even at the time, and was intended to demonstrate their veneration of Jesus.

Botanical family: Santalaceae (sandalwood family)
Extraction method: steam distillation of wood
ORAC: 1.655 μmol TE/100g
Principal components: alpha-santalol, beta-santalol

Sandalwood was used in 19th-century Western medicine to treat chronic bronchitis and all kinds of urological complaints; it also features in ancient writings such as Dioscorides' manual *De Materia medica*, a text that was the standard reference work in the West for the medicinal application of herbs and plants for some 1,700 years. Sandalwood has been valued in India since ancient times as a way of helping people to enter into a state of meditation and prayer and is still applied to the foreheads of Indian monks in the form of a paste. It has a cooling, calming effect on the brain during meditation.

Helping us to switch off from our daily thoughts and worries during meditation, sandalwood oil facilitates immersion in the self while extending and expanding consciousness during meditation. It combines the Kundalini energies of the root and the crown chakras to help us feel properly grounded and connected to what lies above, an important prerequisite for meditation. The application of the oil can refine the perception of subtle energies over time.

Genuine sandalwood comes from a semiparasitic evergreen tree that is native to Southern Asia. Sandalwood trees tap their hosts' roots for water and nutrients for around the first seven years of growth, but take some forty more years to reach the point at which they can be harvested, by which time they will have reached a height of 40–50ft (12–15m). This is when the tree will produce the highest yield of oil and be able to provide around 440lb (200kg) of wood. Extracting sandalwood essential oil is an extremely laborious undertaking: as well as the requirement for the tree to reach the correct age for harvesting, the oil has to mature for some six months after distillation to develop its full scent. The older the oil, the better the fragrance, hence its high price.

Attar of roses (rose otto) essential oil is produced in India using a special process in which rose oil is distilled in sandalwood oil and blended to create a richly scented mixture with powerful properties.

Sandalwood is also an endangered species, so its essential oil should be used very sparingly for environmental reasons. Oils with similar suggested uses, such as frankincense, can therefore be used in place of sandalwood.

PROPERTIES

Sandalwood was valued in popular medicine for the following properties:

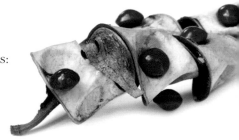

- expectorant
- antibacterial
- antispasmodic
- combats insomnia
- soothes the skin
- removes "false" programming from cell memory

Warning: Do not use sandalwood essential oil if suffering from nephritis.

Sandalwood essential oil contains very high levels of sesquiterpenes (approximately 90 percent). These help to increase the intake of oxygen, particularly to the brain, ensuring a better supply to cerebral glands such as the pineal and pituitary glands. Sandalwood oil can support the endocrine system as a whole. It also contains substances similar to the male hormone androgen, along with compounds that can have a regulatory effect on the womb.

The oil can lift the mood and/or have euphoria-inducing (euphorogenic) and aphrodisiac effects. It helps to sharpen the memory, boosts the immune system, and is useful as a general tonic, with strengthening and invigorating effects both physically and mentally.

Sandalwood oil can have a positive, stimulating effect on the amygdala, a paired structure in the limbic system of the brain that is closely connected with our emotions. Its tasks essentially include analysing danger and assessing situations in preparation for a response. The amygdala helps to activate our vital defensive reactions. Sandalwood essential oil sensitizes our inner warning system so that we can react appropriately to situations in daily life.

POSSIBLE APPLICATIONS

Given that sandalwood has become a scarce resource, ensure it is used sustainably and inhale its scent directly from the vial.

Daily exercise
If you find switching off from the worries of daily life challenging or getting to sleep difficult, try inhaling the scent of sandalwood essential oil directly from the vial. You should begin to experience a sense of calm as your thoughts quieten and settle, and peace returns to your mind.

Frankincense

(Boswellia cateri)

Song of Solomon 3:6
"Who is this that cometh out of the wilderness like pillars of smoke, perfumed with myrrh and frankincense, with all powders of the merchants?"

FRANKINCENSE IN HISTORY

The use of frankincense essential oil dates back 5,000 years and is well documented in historical sources. It is also known as olibanum or "oil of Lebanon." In the days when frankincense was more valuable than gold (due to its various properties, it was used to treat many illnesses), the Three Wise Men (Magi) from the East brought Jesus gifts of gold, frankincense, and myrrh on his birth. Only the rich could afford the oil made from its resin.

The frankincense tree can withstand the extreme heat and aridity of a desert. Workers risk their lives when harvesting the resin since a species of venomous snake habitually lives in the areas where the trees grow. Like myrrh, frankincense is harvested from a species of *Burseraceae*, the incense tree family. In the same way that sap is tapped from the maple tree in order to make syrup, deep cuts are made in the trunk of the frankincense tree, releasing a white resinous substance. Once dried, it falls to the floor in small lumps and is collected.

Since ancient times, many different cultures have made use of frankincense, principally for religious purposes. The Phoenicians living along the eastern coast of the Mediterranean Sea are thought to have secured a monopoly on its trade for a considerable length of time. Frankincense was a part of people's lives from the moment of their birth to their death: it was used to anoint the head of a newborn baby to calm it after birth and for many different ailments, such as to promote the healing of broken bones, as an antidote to poison, and to treat those suffering from cholera and abdominal or chest pains. Virtually every known disease was treated with frankincense.

As a so-called "stairway to heaven," the essential oil was also used to help ease the passage of the dying and the final release of the soul. Frankincense was seen as a protective oil for worshipers of the Egyptian god Nefertem, the god of warriors as well as of salves, anointing oils, and scents. It was also burned and ground to a powder to be used as kohl, the black eyeliner favored by ancient Egyptians, while in China rejuvenating masks made from a paste containing frankincense powder would be applied to the skin.

Botanical family: Burseraceae (incense tree family)

Extraction method: steam distillation from resin

ORAC: 630 μmol TE/100g

Principal components: alpha-pinene, limonene, sabinene, myrcene, beta-caryophyllene, alpha-thujene, incensole

PROPERTIES

Frankincense was valued in popular medicine for the following properties:

- antiseptic
- anti-inflammatory
- enhances mood
- muscle relaxant
- regenerates cells
- boosts the immune system

Frankincense has a calming effect on the mind and so assists in meditation and recuperation after a challenging day. It enhances sensitive perception and opens the gates to the subtle, higher world, reinforcing feelings of devotion.

Unlike the other Bible oils, frankincense essential oil contains only minor levels of sesquiterpenes (8–11 percent), but it shares their positive effects by increasing oxygen levels in the blood and cells, and improving the blood supply to the pituitary gland and hypothalamus. It also contains monoterpenes, which help to promote normal cell growth and have protective, antioxidant properties.

Frankincense is prized in the perfume industry both for its exotic scent and its qualities as a powerful base oil.

POSSIBLE APPLICATIONS

The essential oil has a calming effect when applied to the forehead (remember to dilute it with a carrier oil for sensitive skin). It can also be applied to the chakra points or foot reflex zones, inhaled from between the palms of the cupped hands, or nebulized in an ultrasonic diffusor, and can help to cleanse and purify the air when used as a room spray or in an ultrasonic diffusor.

Uses in energetic protection
The oil provides good protection for the aura. For example, it can help to build up a personal protection field for therapists who are in contact with their clients physically during treatment. Apply 1 drop to the heart chakra and also massage it into the nape of the neck. This will boost the energy field of the person applying the oil and help to protect them from the absorption of external energies.

Daily exercise
To counteract having absorbed any undesirable energy, try this recipe for a cleansing bath. Mix 10–15 drops of frankincense essential oil in 2 teaspoons of honey (or a handful of alkali salt/sodium bicarbonate or 1.5fl oz/50ml of chemical-free skin cream) and add it to your bathwater. As you relax in the water, think about washing away any energies that are not good for you, releasing you from unhealthy habits and connections. You should feel deeply cleansed after bathing.

Hyssop

(Hyssopus officinalis)

Exodus 12:22

"And ye shall take a bunch of hyssop, and dip it in the blood that is in the bason, and strike the lintel and the two side posts with the blood that is in the bason; and none of you shall go out at the door of his house until the morning."

Psalm 51:7

"Purge me with hyssop, and I shall be clean: wash me, and I shall be whiter than snow."

HYSSOP IN HISTORY

Hyssop has long been much prized for its antiseptic properties. The Greeks called it *hyssopos*, a term derived from the Hebrew word *ezob*, meaning something similar to "pleasant-smelling herb." This hardy plant originates in Southern Europe and was brought to the West by the Romans, eventually reaching America with early settlers. It can be found growing wild in France, generally near lavender or rosemary. The strong scent attracts butterflies and bees, and its nectar creates a rich and aromatic honey.

Because of its purifying and disinfectant properties, hyssop was also used to ward off the plague. Its powerful cleansing effect is attributable to its ketone levels of around 50 percent.

Hyssop is mentioned in the Bible as part of the celebration of Passover (see the Bible passage at the beginning of this section), and Numbers 19:6 reveals that it was also used in cleansing rituals. It is also referenced in Psalm 51:7. A branch of hyssop with a sponge soaked in vinegar was held out to Jesus on the cross to quench his thirst, as in John 19:29–30, where we read: "Now there was set a vessel full of vinegar: and they filled a sponge with vinegar, and put it upon hyssop, and put it to his mouth. When Jesus therefore had received the vinegar, he said It is finished: and he bowed his head, and gave up the ghost."

The Romans valued hyssop for its aphrodisiac properties and added it to dishes that also included thyme, pepper, and ginger. Greek physicians Galen (circa 130–200 CE) and Dioscorides (circa 40–90 CE) both praised its expectorant effects, while herbalist and polymath Hildegard of Bingen boiled it in honey as a treatment for strengthening the lungs. The sap of the plant was also applied to the face as a toner. Books of Chinese medicine claim that hyssop is beneficial for the lungs, the nervous system, and the mind while also boosting the immune system. It has been grown as a culinary herb in France since the Middle Ages, where it is added to game and poultry dishes to balance out fats and ease the digestive process.

Due to its high levels of pinocamphone, hyssop essential oil can have toxic effects, so use it with extreme caution. Always dilute it with a neutral

Botanical family: Lamiaceae
or *Labiatae* (deadnettle family)
Extraction method: steam
distillation of branches and leaves
ORAC: 20.900 µmol TE/100g
Principal components:
limese, beta-pinene, sabinene,
pinocamphone, gemacrene D,
iso-pinochamphone

carrier oil when applying it to the body, but it is much safer to inhale its scent instead.

From a spiritual perspective, hyssop is an effective oil for cleansing a room. Use it to remove energies that may interfere with the atmosphere of a room being prepared for meditation or therapy, for example. For personal use, it helps to break up tension auras caused by an overworked mind, when thoughts keep going around in endless circles.

Ambitious people who put a lot of pressure on themselves may find some relief with the oil when they realize that these pressures are self-imposed. It will help them to take a step back and see things from a calmer perspective.

PROPERTIES

Hyssop was valued in popular medicine for the following properties:

- antiseptic
- antibacterial
- antiviral
- antispasmodic
- digestive
- anthelmintic (antiparasitic)
- helps to heal wounds
- regulates lipometabolism (metabolism of fats and other lipids)

Hyssop oil stimulates creativity and aids meditation. People either love or hate its scent. If you find it unpleasant, it may be an indication of emotional blockages. In addition to its cleansing effects on a physical level, hyssop essential oil also brings profound clarity mentally and emotionally. The oil can help to reduce excessive feelings of guilt as well.

POSSIBLE APPLICATIONS

If the oil is to be used on the body, it must first be diluted with equal parts of a neutral carrier oil and then applied to the desired area, such as the chakra points or the foot reflex zones. Its scent can also be inhaled from between cupped hands or directly from the vial, and/or nebulized in an ultrasonic diffusor.

- Apply 1 drop of diluted hyssop oil to the intestine reflex zone on the foot, and massage it in with a gentle pressure. The oil will release any blocked energy in the digestive tract and help to carry away any toxins trapped in the body.

- Apply 1 drop of diluted hyssop oil to the shoulders to help relieve emotional burdens.

- Apply 1 drop of diluted hyssop oil to the lung reflex zone on the foot to relieve feelings of anxiety and worry.

- A drop of diluted hyssop oil applied to the throat around the area of the larynx helps us to process suppressed emotions and can clear the throat chakra.

Daily exercise

If a room feels tainted by unstable and troubling emotions such as anger caused by conflict or depression, add 1–2 drops of hyssop essential oil to a spray bottle full of water and mist the room with this mixture. Note how the energies change. Hyssop is a very effective spiritual cleanser that is useful to keep to hand in this way.

Cedarwood, Atlas

(Cedrus atlantica)

1 Kings 9:10–11

"And it came to pass at the end of twenty years, when Solomon had built the two houses, the house of the Lord, and the king's house, (*Now* Hiram the king of Tyre had furnished Solomon with cedar trees and fir trees, and with gold, according to all his desire,) that then king Solomon gave Hiram twenty cities in the land of Galilee."

CEDARWOOD IN HISTORY

The cedar family includes various species of long-lived coniferous evergreens. These include the Atlas (or silver) cedar, which is native to the Atlas Mountains of Morocco, and the Lebanese cedar, which still grows in Syria and Southern Turkey. Another species of cedar is native to Cyprus, while the Himalayan cedar grows in part of this famous mountain range. The Atlas and Lebanese cedars are the closest genetically, although only the Himalayan and Atlas cedars are still used to produce essential oil today. The scent of the oil from the Lebanese cedar must have been particularly attractive, as

Botanical family: Pinaceae
(pine family)
Extraction method: steam
distillation of bark
ORAC: 169,000 µmol TE/100g
Principal components: alpha-
himachalene, beta-himachalene,
gamma-himachalene, delta-
cadinene

centuries ago perfumers were effusive in their descriptions of its fragrance. However, oil is no longer manufactured from the Lebanese cedar and the tree has been a protected species for some time now.

Cedarwood essential oil was already being extracted more than 6,000 years ago (it has been found among grave goods in the pyramids of Egypt), and as a result it is one of the oldest known essential oils in human history. A number of different cultures, from the Egyptians to the Tibetans, especially prized the cedar, and the wood is used even today in Tibetan medicine and to aid meditation.

The cedar is also the tree species most often mentioned in the Bible, symbolizing fertility and wealth. With its physical majesty and harmonizing properties, it is the tree of kings, and thanks to its links to spirituality was often used as a building material for temples— the mighty cedars of Lebanon were used to build King Solomon's temple, for example. The tree represents immortality, while the scent of the wood promotes clear thinking. Solomon was probably initiated into the effects of essential oils and made use of this knowledge during his reign as the scent of the cedar was ubiquitous in his palaces. The wood is rich in essential oils and also repels insects and pests.

Cedarwood oil was used in conjunction with the oils of myrrh and sandalwood for the embalming procedure in ancient Egypt due to its insecticide and antimicrobial properties. It was also used in Egyptian cosmetics as a tonic for the skin and was prized for its calming properties. The Greek physicians Galen and Dioscorides describe *cedrium* as a resin that protects against decay, and in India the oil was used in cleansing rituals. It was also used to improve lymph flow, to regenerate the arteries, and to treat skin conditions and tuberculosis.

Leviticus 14 contains a law for the cleansing of lepers and houses. A ritual for lepers describes using cedarwood, hyssop, scarlet (carmine), and the blood of two freshly slaughtered birds (Leviticus 14:4) so that the sick person may be reintroduced into the community. After eight days, a further ritual was conducted, during which a massage rite was carried out using olive oil and the blood of another sacrificial animal, and the leper was anointed with oil on the earlobe, thumb, and the big toe. "And the priest shall take some of the blood of the trespass offering and the priest shall put it upon the tip of the right ear of him that is to be cleansed, and upon the thumb of his right hand, and upon the great toe of his right foot." (Leviticus 14:14) The areas of the body mentioned are each connected with special reflex zones that help to resolve blockages. This technique was intended to remove the "impurity" from the sufferer and to make relations between the sufferer and God pure once more.

Writing in 1698, French chemist Nicolas Lémery (1645–1750) describes how cedarwood resin has therapeutic properties as an antiseptic for the urinary tract and the lungs. Cedarwood oil is still used as a base in the perfume industry today, where it is principally employed in the manufacture of fragrances for men.

PROPERTIES

Cedarwood was valued in popular medicine for the following
properties:

- antibacterial
- antispasmodic
- disinfectant
- antifungal
- expectorant
- calms the nerves
- reduces stress
- boosts circulation
- invigorates the respiratory organs
- stimulates lymphatic function
- promotes blood flow

Cedar has the highest levels of sesquiterpenes of any plant (98 percent). The essential oil stabilizes the beta and theta frequencies of the brain waves, and can help us to remain focused and work toward achieving our desired outcome in important business meetings. It can also boost self-esteem. The essential oil has a restabilizing effect after a period of intense effort, delivers harmony and strength on both a physical and emotional level, and helps overanalytical minds to relax. It also helps to resolve emotional tension and aggression. When combined with lavender oil, cedarwood intensifies the experience even more.

Warning: Cedarwood oil is unsuitable if you are pregnant or epileptic, and it should not be used for children.

The oil of visionaries. It encourages us to dream again, to hold on to those dreams and make them come true. The cedar contains male phytohormones (plant hormones) and promotes their harmonization. Many men find this scent very pleasant. The oil can also be sexually stimulating. Mixed with a little carrier oil, it can be applied after shaving or used as a deodorant.

Practical tip: Take a clean glass jar, add the carrier oil, and heat it over a small candle. Once the oil is pleasantly warm, add the cedarwood oil and apply the mixture.

Warning: Take care not to allow the oil to get too hot.

POSSIBLE APPLICATIONS

For a sensual massage

Cedarwood essential oil can strengthen erotic attraction. To treat a partner to a sensual massage, add rose, cedarwood, and ylang ylang oils to a little warm carrier oil, apply to the skin, and massage in.

For personal well-being

For a particularly relaxing massage when you have the time to fully enjoy its effects, gently warm 2 teaspoons of carrier oil and add 3 drops of essential cedarwood oil. Rub the combined oils into the soles of your feet, the palms of your hands, and your face. This should be a deeply relaxing experience and is even more pleasant if a partner is able to massage you with the oil.

Be kind to your skin and bathe in water to which cedarwood oil has been added. Mix 10–15 drops of the oil in 1.5fl oz (50ml) of chemical-free skin cream (or 2 teaspoons of honey or a handful of alkali salt/sodium bicarbonate) and add it to your bathwater for soft skin.

Daily use

Energize 1 drop of cedarwood oil in your hand (see p. 90) with a little carrier oil and apply it to your forehead (on your third eye). The scent can also be inhaled from between the cupped palms of your hands or nebulized in an ultrasonic diffusor.

The essential oil can also be applied to the chakras or worked into the reflex zones of the feet. An added benefit is that it helps to keep moths at bay. Aromatic cedarwood balls are available for this purpose (try adding a drop of cedarwood oil to make them even more effective). Place several in your wardrobe to keep your clothes moth-free.

On a practical level, cedar yields large amounts of oil, making the finest quality cedarwood oil particularly good value for money.

Daily exercise

Apply 1 drop of cedarwood oil to your forehead before an important appointment and inhale the scent. Visualize how you would like the meeting to go. We wish you every success!

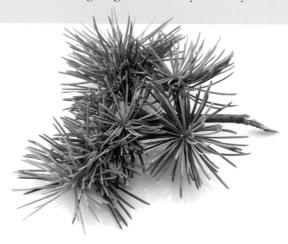

Cistus

(Cistus ladanifer/labdanum)

Genesis 37:25

"And they sat down to eat bread: and they lifted up their eyes and looked, and behold, a company of Ishmaelites came from Gilead with their camels bearing spicery and balm [the resin of the gum rockrose/cistus] and myrrh, going to carry it down to Egypt."

CISTUS IN HISTORY

Cistus is also known as gum rockrose or labdanum. It grows on barren, stony soil and as a member of the mallow family is quite different from the garden roses with which we are all familiar. In warm environments, the resin of cistus is exuded from the plant like small drops of sweat and collects on the plant's leaves.

Centuries ago, goatherds would drive their flocks through gum rockrose bushes and the viscous resin would stick to the animals' coats. It was then either combed or cut out and boiled, after which the precious resin would float to the surface. A later technique involved dragging strips of leather through the bushes to collect the resin. It was popular combined with frankincense in churches.

The use of gum rockrose in Egypt dates back as far as the 4th century BCE. In Greece, to relax after a difficult day and to reinvigorate and boost the immune system, it was made into a tea that was drunk all year round. Midwives would also use it to bathe wounds acquired during childbirth and to support their healing. Gum rockrose was particularly prized as a treatment for injuries to the skin thanks to its property of promoting cell regeneration—rather like a sticking plaster in liquid form!

Botanical family: Cistaceae (cistus family)
Extraction method: steam distillation of leaves and branches
ORAC: 38.648 µmol TE/100g
Principal components: alpha-pinene, camphene, bornyl acetate, trans-pinocarveole

Gum rockrose is referred to as labdanum in the Bible, meaning a fragrant resin. It is mentioned in Genesis 37:25 and 43:11 as "balm."

PROPERTIES

Cistus essential oil was valued in popular medicine for the following properties:

- antibacterial
- antiviral
- antifungal
- anti-inflammatory
- promotes wound healing
- boosts the immune system

Gum rockrose has a balancing and stabilizing effect and helps to lift the mood. The scent penetrates deep into the consciousness, and on a spiritual level promotes awareness of the individual self. Its scent has also been used since ancient times to stimulate visions and help in the search for meaning in life.

The plant is rich in polyphenols (tannins) and resins, which can have a positive effect on the elimination of heavy metals from the body. As a study of heavy smokers carried out by the University of Lübeck in Germany demonstrated, cadmium levels in the blood dropped considerably when the test subjects drank a daily decoction of gum rockrose tea for a period of four weeks.

POSSIBLE APPLICATIONS

Cistus is one of the base oils used in perfume manufacture and improves the bonding of scents to the skin, which affects the longevity of a perfume.

Try a bath enriched with cistus essential oil to promote relaxation. Add 10–15 drops of cistus oil to 1.5fl oz (50ml) of chemical-free skin cream (or 2 teaspoons of honey or a handful of alkali salt/sodium bicarbonate), combine them and add to the bathwater.

The oil can also be used as a room spray. Fill a small spray bottle with distilled water and add 5–10 drops of cistus essential oil per 1.5fl oz (50ml) of water, depending on the required intensity of scent. Spray the mixture around the room to create a pleasant atmosphere.

Cistus essential oil is extremely suitable for applying to the chakras or the reflex zones of the foot. It can also be nebulized or inhaled from between the cupped palms of the hands.

Daily exercise
Cistus essential oil can help in meditation. Take a drop of oil, energize it (see p. 90), and breathe the scent in deeply through your nose. Follow your usual meditation routine, taking care to note any images or insights that may come to you.

Cypress

(Cupressus)

Isaiah 60:13

"The glory of Lebanon shall come unto thee,
the fir tree, the pine tree, and the box [cypress]
together to beautify the place of my sanctuary;
and I will make the place of my feet glorious."

CYPRESS IN HISTORY

The ancient Egyptians were familiar with cypress essential oil and its uses and documented their findings on papyrus scrolls. They would also use the wood of the cypress tree to make coffins for the dead, while the Phoenicians and Cretans used it to build ships and make

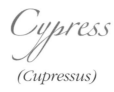

bows. Icons depicting gods were carved from cypress wood in Greece, where the tree was sacred to Hades, god of the underworld.

Known as the tree of light and eternity, the cypress offers us a connection between heaven and Earth, its tall columnar form both rooted in the ground and pointing upward toward the sky. It is therefore no surprise to learn that cypresses are frequently found in churchyards to symbolize eternal life. The portal of St. Peter's Basilica in Rome is made of cypress wood and shows no sign of rot or decay, even after 1,200 years.

Both male and female flowers grow on some species of the tree and the oil contains high levels of monoterpenes, which intercept and trap free radicals and repair DNA in the body.

Botanical family: Cupressaceae (cypress family)

Extraction method: steam distillation of branches

ORAC: 24.300 µmol TE/100g

Principal components: monoterpenes, alpha-pinene, beta-pinene, delta-3-carene, limese, cedrole, myrcene, manoyle oxide, isopimaradiene, karahanaenone

PROPERTIES

Cypress essential oil was valued in popular medicine for the following properties.

* antibacterial
* anti-infectious
* antispasmodic
* cleanses the lymph
* improves lymphatic flow
* boosts the liver
* helps to ease water retention
* promotes blood flow
* helps alleviate chilblains and varicose veins

- contains female phytohormones (plant hormones) and so helps to rebalance the hormonal system in women

- kind to the skin, helps to heal scars

Recent studies have demonstrated the oil's antimicrobial properties and its effect on the biofilm, the mucus layer that many bacteria form to protect themselves but which can induce inflammation in the host and cause harm. Cypress essential oil can destroy this biofilm.

The oil has a stabilizing and grounding effect in times of stress, such as when professional life is particularly challenging or when moving house, as well as during periods of transition, such as the end of life process, when the oil provides support for both the person involved and their relatives. It helps us to process and deal with emotional trauma and is also particularly effective for alleviating physical stress.

Here's a familiar situation. One moment everything is pleasant and going well, life is just as it should be and you are confident things will stay as they are—then suddenly, with a bang, life has a surprise in store for you. Cypress oil can provide great support when some form of change or disruption is afoot.

It helps us to accept change, to negotiate, and let go of situations.

- Acceptance, in this case, means recognizing a problem/topic/ situation/challenge for what it is and no longer working against it; it means no longer feeling regret about things that you cannot change.

- Negotiation, in this respect, involves reorienting yourself to deal with a situation and daring to take steps in a new direction.

- Letting go is about not clinging on to something but instead being able to set it free again.

In addition, cypress oil can help you to embark upon, persevere with, and complete whatever you decide to undertake, so it is a very useful oil during times of change.

> **Warning:** Cypress essential oil is not suitable for pregnant women or people with epilepsy.

POSSIBLE APPLICATIONS

Cypress essential oil can have aphrodisiac properties, but the following combination will bring calm and restraint to a particularly stormy relationship, should this be necessary: mix sandalwood, cypress, and bergamot oils with a little warm carrier oil, apply it to your partner's body, and massage it in.

Energetic cleansing
We absorb not only prana (subtle life force energy) through the spleen chakra but also "vampires" from the higher plane that sap our vitality. If you feel drained or lacking in energy after visiting certain places—perhaps a nursing home, hospital, cemetery, a large shopping mall, or just a very busy location—try the following:

Combine a drop of cypress essential oil with a little carrier oil and energize this mixture (see p. 90). Now apply it to your skin, just below your ribcage on the left side of the body and to your back around the kidney area. Imagine your hands as light sabers, severing any threads through which your energy is being drained.

You might also like to experiment with vocalization as you perform these energetic separations.

Cypress essential oil can also be applied to the reflex zones of the feet, inhaled from between the cupped hands, or nebulized in an ultrasonic diffusor.

Daily exercise

After a particularly exhausting day, perhaps one that you have spent entirely on your feet, or if your legs feel tired or swollen, try this application: mix 1–2 drops of cypress essential oil with a little neutral carrier oil, and apply it to your legs and the soles of your feet, and massage in gently. And if you can then relax and put your feet up, so much the better. Enjoy!

ALTERNATIVE OILS

Due to environmental factors and overharvesting, some plants have steadily been acquiring protected status in recent years, hence my belief in the importance of working with producers of essential oils who respect and treat the natural world with care rather than being guided by short-term profit.

Spikenard and galbanum are two such endangered species. The use of these protected plants is now forbidden throughout the entire essential oil industry. It was a sad day indeed when these soothing oils ceased to be available. The absence of their vibrational effects would certainly be noticed in the "raindrop energy treatment" for example (see p. 90). As a result, we have researched alternative oils with vibrations that come close to those of spikenard and galbanum and so can recommend vetiver and elemi.

Vetiver
(Vetiveria zizaniodes)

Vetiver essential oil offers an alternative to spikenard. Vetiver oil is fairly viscous, therefore to help it flow more easily, place a vial of the oil somewhere warm for a few minutes just before it is due to be applied. This could simply be in a pocket, where the warmth of your body will warm the oil just enough to ensure a smoother flow.

The scent of vetiver is earthy and the smell of the root is quite noticeable. When applying the oil topically, I am always powerfully aware of just how deeply the recipient enters a state of relaxation. When

Botanical family: Poaceae
(bunchgrass family)
Extraction method: steam
distillation of the root
Principal components:
isovalencenol, khusimol,
alpha-vetivone, beta-vetivone,
beta-vetivenes

combined with cedarwood and lavender, it can also maximize the enjoyment of deep relaxation and help with getting to sleep. Dr. Terry S. Friedmann carried out a study using vetiver, cedarwood, and lavender oils, for patients with ADHD (Attention Deficit and Hyperactivity Disorder). He established that these three essential oils can achieve similar results to synthetic medication but without the side effects. See: http://www.isbewonders .com/wp-content/uploads/2017/05/ADHD -Research-by-Dr.-Terry-Friedmann-1.pdf

The quality of time as we experience it in these first decades of the 21st century brings quite profound anxiety to many people, whether for health-related, economic, or political reasons. Vetiver is very helpful in this respect thanks to the deeply grounding qualities of the oil that is extracted from its root. Trauma can also be managed effectively with vetiver.

The oil is easy to apply in pure or diluted form via a roll-on, to the wrists, nape of the neck, or temples, for example. To boost its grounding effects, apply a drop to the soles of the feet. Due to its wonderfully relaxing properties, we recommend application just before going to bed to induce a good night's sleep.

Elemi

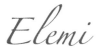

(Canarium luzonicum)

Our search for an alternative to galbanum led us to elemi. The tree from which it is extracted is mostly found in the Philippines. It can grow to a height of up to 100ft (30m) and is tapped by making cuts in the trunk in order to extract the resin in a similar way to frankincense. To close up the wound, the tree produces gum resin, which is then collected and dried out. The small resin lumps can either be burned as incense or processed into essential oil via steam distillation.

The use of elemi stretches back millennia, when the Egyptians would employ it in the embalming process, and its powerful antiseptic properties were also highly prized. Elemi has also been used in Europe for hundreds of years, especially to treat wounds. A special ointment was developed by a 17th century physician to help heal the injuries of wounded soldiers.

Elemi's active ingredients support cleansing and clarification, hence it is frequently used to set the mood before meditation. Its fragrance delivers a sense of optimism and excitement at new beginnings, and it can instill feelings of hope in challenging times.

Elemi's active components are also effective in skin care and in the treatment of scars.

Much like frankincense, regular use of elemi has proved its

Botanical family: Burseraceae (incense tree family)

Extraction method: steam distillation of the gum resin

Principal components: limonene, alpha-phellandrene, sabinene, elemol worth in the battle against wrinkles. Incorporate a drop of elemi into your daily natural skin care routine, both in the morning and evening. Encourage its nurturing active ingredients by tapping the skin gently with your fingertips during application.

Elemi honey mask

A honey mask cleanses the skin and can be made even more effective with a few drops of elemi essential oil. Stir 2 drops of elemi oil into just 1 teaspoon of honey.

In order to open up the pores of the face before applying the mask, fill a bowl with steaming water and add a drop of elemi or frankincense oil (optional). Keeping your face at a comfortable distance from the water in the bowl, cover your head with a towel to trap the steam. Take care not to scald yourself.

After around 3 to 5 minutes, remove the bowl, dry your face, and apply the honey mixture. For a more intense treatment, massage your skin by pinching it with your fingers.

Please note that the honey mask is very sticky, but it is effective. The honey absorbs the toxins that build up on the skin every day and the pinch massage stimulates circulation. Wash the honey mask off with lukewarm water and a clean cloth after approximately 15–20 minutes.

Most people find their skin is soft, silky, and cleansed after the treatment. Should you choose to apply argan oil after the facial, try adding a drop of elemi or frankincense into the oil before applying it topically.

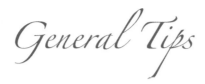

General Tips

This is where our journey together through the world of essential oils from the dawn of history to today finally ends. The more we have learned about these plants and their oils and the myriad uses to which they can be put, and the more we have discovered about the wealth of knowledge that existed even in ancient times, the more consciously we will be able to use these precious substances ourselves today.

These highly therapeutic oils are now readily available, no longer the exclusive preserve of kings and priests, but we would encourage you to work with them in a sustainable and sensible manner since many plants are already threatened with extinction. Therefore, when possible, use the oils in diluted form or by inhaling the scent directly from the vial.

Since applying these oils to the body is also such a pleasurable experience, it is easy to get carried away, but we recommend bearing in mind the scarcity of some and using them carefully and with economy. To create a blend of all the oils, simply add a drop of each to some neutral carrier oil (such as coconut oil) in a 0.5fl oz (20ml) vial. Apply a little of the oil as a foot massage for a great way to start or finish the day and boost your mental and physical energies.

After applying oil to the skin, for the best results, allow it to soak into the skin for around ten minutes and then take a warm shower. This will enable the oil to be fully absorbed by the skin and to penetrate deeper into the tissue. It is natural to feel energized afterwards since many of the oils have the effect of encouraging the uptake of oxygen into the cells of the body. Your skin will feel supple and soft after its application. In the "raindrop energy treatment," drops of herbal oil are dripped liked drops of rain onto the back and then gently massaged into the skin to cleanse bacteria and viruses from the tissue around the spinal area.

A final tip

We have also been able to visibly gauge the effects of the oils by using devices that measure auras, chakras, and energetic organs. The measuring devices reveal an immediate enhancing and harmonizing effect when the oils are energized and the subject recites a prayer or focuses their mind on positive, healthy thoughts. This demonstrates to us how oils and prayer mutually reinforce one another. When oils are applied with positive thoughts in the mind, their vibrational level is even more heightened. Prayer and oils do not have to go hand in hand, and can, of course, be used individually, but when combined, something special may occur. Just try it for yourself!

Energizing oil

Place a little carrier oil in the palm of your left hand and add a drop of essential oil. Now combine the two by rubbing the mixture clockwise around the palm of your left hand with the index and middle finger of your right hand, three times.

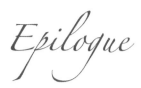

Epilogue

We have observed and filmed the effects of classic and Bible oils on blood, both before and after an application, using darkfield microscopy, a special technique used to examine blood samples.

Observing a classic oil application is like watching a small war being waged in the body, during which the antioxidant effect of the oil sets about eliminating the harmful bacteria. When the Bible oils were applied, the platelets soon lit up and a glowing corona formed around each small blood cell. Blood circulation improved and the immune system became significantly more active.

Anyone can learn to use this technique, no training or qualifications are necessary, and it is equally suitable for interested amateurs to use at home as it is for professionals. The authors regularly offer workshops on the technique.

One particular observation made with a Biopulsar Reflexograph® reading was how the essential oil is directed to the location requiring harmonization. We used cypress essential oil in our experiment. In a test subject focusing on the pelvic region, the organs were very balanced beforehand from a resonance perspective, which remained the case, although the device also revealed small, jagged patterns around the pelvic region. The test subject then confirmed that he did have problems in the pelvic area, so the essential oil had targeted the relevant point. Following the application of another oil that specifically supports the joints, the jagged pattern transformed into small waves. This process was very exciting to watch.

With reference to the aura images, we could observe how tiny red tongues of fire shot through the aura when cassia was used, and the subject also felt very warm. We also saw how electromagnetic pollution can collapse the energy field and how oils were able to restore its stability.

These were not scientific investigations but experiments to satisfy our personal thirst for knowledge. There was no room to include the images in this small book, but it is much more interesting to have your own before/after pictures taken.

We would be delighted if we have tempted you to become interested in using essential oils. It is a blessing that they are now available for everyone to explore and use, and we hope you enjoy your own experiences.

We are happy to answer any questions you may have.

Karin Opitz-Kreher and Johannes Huber

Acknowledgments

We would like to offer our special thanks to all those who have taught us (knowingly or otherwise!) so much about oils in various seminars and conversations over recent years.

We would also like to thank Beate and Janine for their expert support in Bible knowledge.

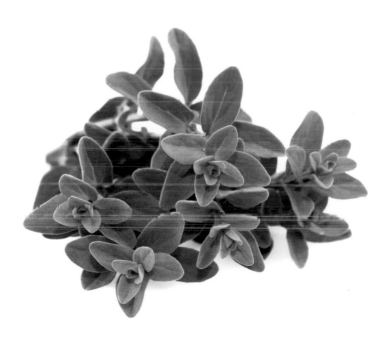

Bibliography

Price, Shirley. *Practical Aromatherapy: How to use essential oils to restore health and vitality.* Thorsons, London. 2000.

Stewart, Dr. David Stewart & Holger Grimme. *Healing Oils of the Bible.* Care Publications, 2003.

Young, D. Gary. *Essential Oils, Integrative Medical Guide.* Life Science Publishing, Orem, 2013.

Young, D. Gary. *Essential Oils, Pocket Reference.* Life Science Publishing, Orem, 2014.

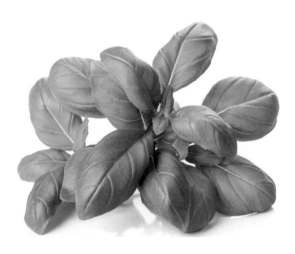

About the Authors

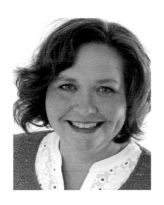

Karin Opitz-Kreher is trained in Aura-Soma, Aura-Soma bodywork, and foot reflexology harmonization. She also works as a meditation group leader following Ralph Jordan and as a biofeedback therapist, using the SCIO system for stress reduction and system harmonization. She discovered the world of essential oils in 2013 and has been making use of the traditional knowledge of oils in her work ever since. Karin also gives seminars on their use in energy work.

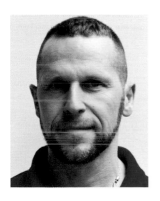

Johannes Huber is an alternative practitioner whose interest in essential oils goes back to his youth. He has been working with them in aromatherapy and in the care of the sick and elderly for more than ten years. The focus of his work also includes darkfield microscopy diagnosis.

Picture Credits

Pages 1, 5: nito (flacon) and photo-oasis (Bible); pp. 6, 33, 45: Diana Taliun; pp. 8, 69: jopelka; pp. 9, 78: Steve Photography; p. 11: Only Fabrizio; p. 12: eldeiv; pp. 14, 18, 31: Madlen; p. 17: Sandra van der Steen; p. 19: LanKS; pp. 20, 41, 59: marilyn barbone; p. 22: Alexander Raths; p. 24: Richard Griffin; p. 27: JIANG HONGYAN; p. 29: Pinci; p. 32: Yongkiet Jitwattanatam; pp. 35, 46, 48, 93: Scisetti Alfio; p. 37: Henrik Larsson; p. 42: unpict; pp. 50, 86: wasanajai; p. 56: KPG-Payless2; p. 60: Swapan Photography; p. 62: spline_x; p. 65: CBasting; p. 67: Morinka; pp. 71, 76: Volosina; p. 73: Maya Morenko; p. 80: Formatoriginal; p. 83: de2marco; p. 88: Glenda Esperida; p. 90: Dionisvera; p. 94: Olga Miltsova. All Shutterstock.com

All Bible quotes are taken from the King James version.

For further information and to request a book catalog contact:
Inner Traditions, One Park Street, Rochester, Vermont 05767

Earthdancer Books is an Inner Traditions imprint
Phone: +1-800-246-8648, customerservice@innertraditions.com
www.earthdancerbooks.com • www.innertraditions.com

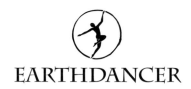

EARTHDANCER

AN INNER TRADITIONS IMPRINT